Prevention in Community Mental Health Centers

The *Prevention in Human Services* series:

- *Helping People to Help Themselves: Self-Help and Prevention*, edited by Leonard D. Borman, Leslie Borck, Robert E. Hess, and Frank L. Pasquale
- *Early Intervention Programs for Infants*, edited by Howard A. Moss, Robert E. Hess, and Carolyn Swift
- ℞ *Television: Enhancing the Preventive Impact of TV*, edited by Joyce Sprafkin, Carolyn Swift, and Robert E. Hess
- *Innovations in Prevention*, edited by Robert E. Hess and Jared A. Hermalin
- *Strategies for Needs Assessment in Prevention*, edited by Alex Zautra, Kenneth Bachrach, and Robert E. Hess
- *Aging and Prevention: New Approaches for Preventing Health and Mental Health Problems in Older Adults*, edited by Sharon Simson, Laura B. Wilson, Jared A. Hermalin, and Robert E. Hess
- *Studies in Empowerment: Steps Toward Understanding and Action*, edited by Julian Rappaport, Carolyn Swift, and Robert E. Hess
- *Prevention: The Michigan Experience*, edited by Betty Tableman and Robert E. Hess
- *Beyond the Individual: Environmental Approaches and Prevention*, edited by Abraham Wandersman and Robert E. Hess
- *The Ecology of Prevention: Illustrating Mental Health Consultation*, edited by James G. Kelly and Robert E. Hess
- *Prevention and Health: Directions for Policy and Practice*, edited by Alfred H. Katz, Jared A. Hermalin, and Robert E. Hess
- *Prevention: Toward a Multidisciplinary Approach*, edited by Leonard A. Jason, Robert E. Hess, Robert D. Felner, and John N. Moritsugu
- *A Guide to Conducting Prevention Research in the Community: First Steps,* by James G. Kelly with the collaboration of Nancy Dassoff, Ira Levin, Janice Schreckengost, Stephen P. Stelzner and B. Eileen Altman
- *The National Mental Health Association: Eighty Years of Involvement in the Field of Prevention*, edited by Robert E. Hess and Jean Delong
- *Protecting the Children: Strategies for Optimizing Emotional and Behavioral Development*, edited by Raymond P. Lorion
- *Prevention in Community Mental Health Centers*, edited by Robert E. Hess and John Morgan

Prevention in Community Mental Health Centers

Robert E. Hess
John Morgan
Editors

The Haworth Press
New York • London

Prevention in Community Mental Health Centers has also been published as *Prevention in Human Services*, Volume 7, Number 2 1990.

The Haworth Press, Inc. 10 Alice Street, Binghamton, NY 13904-1580
EUROSPAN/Haworth, 3 Henrietta Street, London WC2E 8LU England

Library of Congress Cataloging-in-Publication Data

Prevention in community mental health centers : Robert E. Hess, John Morgan, editors.
p. cm.
Has also been published as Prevention in human services, v. 7, no. 2 1990.
Includes bibliographical references.
ISBN 0-86656-999-5 (alk. paper) : $24.95
1. Community mental health services – United States. 2. Mental illness – United States – Prevention. I. Hess, Robert, 1984- . II. Morgan, John, 1948- .
[DNLM: 1. Community Mental Health Centers. 2. Community Psychiatry. 3. Mental Disorders – prevention & control. W1 PR497 v. 7 no. 2 / WM 31.5 P94406]
RA790.6.P74 1990
362.2'2'0973 – dc20
DNLM/DLC
for Library of Congress

90-4418
CIP

Prevention in Community Mental Health Centers

CONTENTS

Introduction 1

Robert E. Hess
John Morgan

Competence Enhancement and Primary Prevention as Core Functions of CMHCs: A Case Study and Blueprint for the Future 3

John F. Clabby
Maurice J. Elias

Stage One: Introduction and Adoption of an Innovation 6
Stage Two: Implementation and Expansion of the Innovation 9
Stage Three: Institutionalization of an Innovation as an Accepted Organizational Entity 11

The Development and Management of Prevention Services Within a Comprehensive, Medical School-Based, Community Mental Health Center 17

Steven W. Godin
Lucille Carr-Kaffashan
Paulette Moore Hines

Historical and Theoretical Considerations 18
History and Phases of Development of Prevention Services, UMDNJ – Community Mental Health Center 25
Overview of Current Prevention Services 38
Conclusion 46

Twenty Years of Primary Prevention: Consultation, Education and Prevention at the Washtenaw County Community Mental Health Center 49
Ruth F. Schelkun

C,E&P Services 52
The Research/Practice Link 60
Management Issues 62
Place in the Organization 62
Funding 63
Staffing 64
Management Information 65
Process Issues 66
Continuity of Administrative Support and Staff Sophistication 66
Broad Community Involvement and Wide Scope of Service 67
Collaborative Relationships and Community Resource Building 68
Cross Training and Systematizing What Works 68
Attitudes, Behaviors, and Personal Characteristics 69
Keeping Up with the Field 70
Disappointments and Difficulties 70
Conclusion 71

Developing Prevention Programming in a Large Nonprofit Service Agency 75
Thomas A. Duke
Eugene S. Urbain

Rationale for Prevention Programming at Wilder 77
Description 80
Conclusion 87

Divorce Workshops: Community Education for a High Risk Population 89
John Kalafat
Maureen Underwood
Nancy Fiedler
William D. Neigher

Needs Assessment and Planning 93
Making It! Series 94

Process Evaluation 98
Epidemiological Stress Data 101
Additional Program Impact 103
Conclusion 105

Maximizing the Potential for Community Self-Help Through Clearinghouse Approaches **109**
Edward J. Madara

Professional Involvement with Self-Help 114
Development of Self-Help Clearinghouses 115
The New Jersey Self-Help Clearinghouse 118
Empowerment versus Enfeeblement 131
Perspectives on Additional Self-Help Trends 132
Conclusion 135

∞ ALL HAWORTH BOOKS & JOURNALS
ARE PRINTED ON CERTIFIED
ACID-FREE PAPER

ABOUT THE EDITORS

Robert E. Hess, PhD, is the Programs Administrator at Riverwood Center, Benton Harbor, Michigan. He has received several national awards for his work in prevention, has published extensively in the field, and has served on and chaired various organizations devoted to furthering the philosophy of prevention. He is currently a board member of the Mental Health Association in Michigan and a member of the Michigan Department of Mental Health Advisory Group on Prevention and Community/Caregiver Services. He is past Chair of the Division of Prevention of the National Council of Community Mental Health Centers. Dr. Hess is editor of *Prevention in Human Services*.

John Morgan, PhD, is Director of Clinical and Prevention Services, Chesterfield Mental Health-Mental Retardation Department in Chesterfield, Virginia. Dr. Morgan has published and lectured extensively to professional groups in the area of primary prevention. He is active in the Division of Community Psychology of the American Psychological Association and is co-editor of that division's newsletter. He was also the first Chairperson of the Prevention Advisory Council in Virginia. Dr. Morgan received his doctorate in clinical psychology from Pennsylvania State University.

Introduction

In the late 1960s and throughout the decade of the 70s, prevention enjoyed a comparatively prominent role in community mental health centers thanks to federal staffing grants. During the early 1980s, these grants ended and prevention services in most centers were reduced, eliminated, or had their resources diverted into clinical programs. Prevention services were vulnerable because they were unable to generate revenue to the same extent as clinical services.

Many centers, however, did not follow the trend and retained, and in some cases—expanded, their prevention efforts. Some states, Michigan being the prime example, continued to be supportive of prevention and provided the funding required by centers to maintain visible prevention efforts.

Recently, there has been evidence that prevention is enjoying a slow resurgence in mental health centers. As an example, Michigan is moving toward the institution of a prevention coordinator in all of its mental health centers and has established, through a work group convened by a member of the state legislature, a long-range plan for prevention services in the state. Virginia has also developed a plan and the promise of financial support for increased prevention programming. Other states are following.

This volume provides a very small sample of the prevention efforts in mental health centers throughout the country. What is noteworthy is that, in soliciting contributions for this volume, we discovered other equally good programs in Indiana, Ohio, New Jersey, Virginia, Michigan, Illinois, Alabama, Arkansas, California, New York, and Oregon. Unfortunately, we also discovered that prevention professionals in mental health centers are, in general, much more comfortable in providing services than in writing about them.

In time, we hope that a forum will emerge so that readers can learn about these other efforts. For now, we are proud to be able to feature the excellent work of the authors in this volume.

Robert E. Hess
John Morgan

Competence Enhancement and Primary Prevention as Core Functions of CMHCs: A Case Study and Blueprint for the Future

John F. Clabby
University of Medicine and Dentistry
New Jersey-CMHC at Piscataway

Maurice J. Elias
Rutgers University

SUMMARY. The stages through which an innovation passes on its way toward becoming institutionalized within a host setting are delineated. A historical chronicle is presented of how a social problem solving program, designed as a competence enhancing, primary prevention effort, goes through these stages within the hosting public school system. Additionally, a parallel process is described regarding how the Social Problem Solving Program progressed along a similar route within its parent mental health center on its way to

---

The authors acknowledge the many and special contributions of our collaborating systems, the University of Medicine and Dentistry of New Jersey-CMHC at Piscataway, Rutgers University, a host of independent school systems within the State of New Jersey, and a creative and skilled service delivery and research team. Particular appreciation goes to Gary Lamson, Bill Commins, Thomas Schuyler and Michael Gara. Thanks to Barbara Zak and Patricia Dooley for their careful typing of the manuscript.

Correspondence and requests for reprints can be sent to either John F. Clabby, UMDNJ-CMHC at Piscataway, Social Problem Solving Program, 240 Stelton Road, Piscataway, NJ 08854-3248 or Maurice J. Elias, Department of Psychology, Tillett Hall, Rutgers University, New Brunswick, NJ 08903.

becoming a regular and permanent service delivery entity within the mental health center.

Envision a time when community mental health centers no longer think of prevention services as ancillary or adjunctive to the center's main mission. Imagine an era during which the community mental health center comes to see its role as involving the development, evaluation, and responsible dissemination of technologies for psychosocial enhancement. During such a time, the developmental rights of children and adolescents will be given highest priority and the promotion of sound growth will be viewed as a valid end (Masterpasqua, 1981). Prevention of specific conditions such as substance abuse, delinquency, school drop-out, and teen suicide will be likely outcomes, but not the driving force behind the planning and delivery of enhancement-oriented services.

Is this scenario an optimistic look into the twenty-first century? In actuality, the scenario describes the present arrangements at the University of Medicine and Dentistry of New Jersey-Community Mental Health Center (UMDNJ-CMHC) at Piscataway. A competence enhancement service has come into existence even as a number of CMHCs (community mental health centers) increase their emphasis on medicalized, clinical care to very seriously disturbed clients. And, even as schools increase their emphasis on preparing students in the basic academic area, they are also increasingly receptive to the importance—indeed, the *necessity*—of addressing students' social and affective needs (Elias & Maher, 1983).

As a guide for others who are also committed to helping our organizations and institutions change to better serve others, this paper presents a series of stages along which a new, promising, and innovative program passes on its way to become a permanent part of its host institution. As an example of this process, a history will be related regarding how the Social Problem Solving Program, which is a curriculum-based innovation for competence enhancement and primary and secondary preventions, became a part of a school system. Additionally, the story will be told regarding how this program became institutionalized within its own parent CMHC system as a permanent service delivery unit.

Commins (1986) identified three major stages along which innovations pass to become accepted or routine practice within an organization and it is his work that provides our primary theoretical reference point. During the first stage, staff of the potential host organization learn about the existence of the innovation. If sufficiently intrigued, the staff follows up with further questions and investigation to determine how the innovation works. The goal of the staff of the potential host organization is to determine if there is a possible fit between the potential host organization's mission and what the innovation could provide. If a likely fit exists, the leadership of both the host organization and the innovative program agree to collaborate.

The second stage on the road toward institutionalization commences with the implementation of a pilot program. The innovative program works hard at gaining this foothold of long-term acceptance and stability within the host environment with the leadership team making intelligent and sensitive fine tunings and adjustments of the innovation. The program should be carried out with *visibility*, *persistence*, and a generative procedure which encourages *formative monitoring* of the program's implementation, *summative evaluation* of its impacts, and importantly, the transformation of that monitoring and evaluation information into specific feedback that becomes integrated as improved program procedures. This continued improvement and self monitoring of how well the innovation is helping the host organization meet its mission is, in effect, an action-research cycle. It is a cycle that is constantly working toward long term acceptance of the innovation by the host organization much as medical professionals check, re-check, and make adjustments of procedures as they work toward the long-term acceptance by the human body of an organ transplant, anticipating some tendencies of the host organism to reject the "intrusion" of the innovation. When outcome successes that meet the mission of the host organization emerge, the desirability for the innovation grows and so does the pressure to expand the innovation within the organization. Leaders of the innovation need to be prepared to responsibly handle the increased demand for services. Finally, during the third stage, the innovation is routinized as a part of the central functioning of the host agency or organization.

STAGE ONE: INTRODUCTION AND ADOPTION OF AN INNOVATION

In our specific case, the Improving Social Awareness-Social Problem Solving (ISA-SPS) Project had its beginnings in 1979. The concern of the CMHC at that time was to improve its relationship with one of the public school systems within its catchment area. The initial concept was that the clinical care offered to children would be improved if closer cooperation between the school system and the CMHC would develop. The primary motivation on the part of the CMHC was to use its consultation and education staff to develop a positive liaison with the school community so that the *major mission* of the outpatient clinic, i.e., psychotherapy with disturbed clients, could be enhanced.

The CMHC psychologist assigned to this task had become aware of the research literature citing the importance of teaching children flexible coping skills (Kendall & Hollan, 1979) and describing social (or interpersonal) cognitive problem solving skills as a set of abilities that mediates the way children and adults adjust to interpersonal situations (Spivack, Platt, & Shure, 1976). The report of the President's Commission on Mental Health in 1978 also suggested the interpersonal cognitive problem solving strategy as a potential cornerstone for preventive services. In addition to the sound research base validating the promise of this approach, there was a growing recognition that critical decision making and problem solving skills are important parts of academic competence, influencing both indices of academic achievement as well as essential "learning to learn" skills.

The skills that were emphasized (and remain emphasized) within the ISA-SPS Project were drawn from the social problem solving literature (Allen & Associates, 1976) and include:

a. A person's *belief* about whether or not he or she will be effective in handling a problem.
b. The self-control and social awareness skills necessary to function in a group or classroom setting.
c. The capacity to "read" the signs of one's own and other's feelings.

d. The extent to which a person can reliably generate goal-directed solutions and anticipate their consequences, and,
e. A person's ability to develop a realistic plan to carry out a good idea and the ability to learn from experience.

The adoption by the public school was enhanced because a gatekeeping elementary principal recognized the happy convergence of several needs that a program of this type could meet. First, with the program's emphasis on developing children's "thinking" skills, he could host a program that aided the main mission of the school system (i.e., academic), as well as the "secondary" mission (cultivating citizenship and social development). Additionally, if the program worked with children toward the end of their elementary school experience, it could mitigate the impact of the stress his students would experience when they dealt with the problems of the middle school years. For both this school system and most school systems in the country, the first year of middle school represents a peak point of psychological referrals (Rutter, 1980) and, consequently, the burdens on middle school and mental health center staff to attend to student, parent, and teacher stress related to this age group are considerable.

With the assurance that the CMHC psychologist would co-lead two social problem solving classes with two teachers, the school system agreed to pilot a fourth grade level program. Out of a recognition of the need for a formative and summative evaluation of the pilot effort, a community/prevention psychologist from a neighboring university's psychology department was added to the team. During the first year's program, the social problem solving steps, i.e., look for signs of different feelings, tell yourself what the problem is, etc., were verbally woven into the class discussion of open-ended social problem stories (Elardo & Cooper, 1977) by the psychologist and teachers.

During the pilot year, the beginnings of a formal, long-term experimental evaluation of the impact of the social problem solving program, using matched no-treatment control classrooms, was begun. While the initial research findings were encouraging, there were other kinds of positive feedback that were even more significant in encouraging the host environment. Specifically, it was the high degree of consumer satisfaction regarding the experience of the social problem solving lessons that was probably more important than any of the research findings in encouraging the school administration to institutionalize the innovation. The children in the pilot classes eagerly looked forward to the lessons and participated fully and enthusiastically. Additionally, they talked about their experiences at home to their parents. The two involved teachers also had similar, highly positive feelings. They would discuss the lessons with their colleagues, and talk about the positive impact which they felt the lessons were having on classroom climate and how the children were getting better able to handle everyday conflicts as a result of the lessons. As positive feedback regarding the program became known in the community, it lead to a demand—from influential parent leaders of children in the control settings—to expand the program to include all of the fourth and fifth grade classes in the district. This was a recommendation that was strongly agreed to by the superintendent of schools, who subsequently came to the Social Problem Solving Program leaders asking for expansion from two to sixteen classes for the following school year.

Because one of the program's developers was present as a consultant for each lesson that was taught during the pilot year, there had been some assurance regarding quality and standards. With the pressure for expansion that accompanied the first year's success came a concern for how to continue quality and standardization when the program would be delivered by sixteen different teachers. A way had to be found whereby there could be some reasonable assurance that all sixteen teachers taught the same content in a quality way, which would also allow the evaluation team to make reasonable assumptions about these classes when compared to control classes. With an eye toward this issue as well as toward a way of adopting the Social Problem Solving Program more securely within the CMHC delivery system, several benchmarks were attained: (a) the project leaders wrote, and the teachers implemented, a highly scripted curriculum (Elias & Clabby, in press, a) which went a great way toward assuring quality and standardization; (b) funding was obtained from the local school setting; and (c) the consulting CMHC psychologist was encouraged and sanctioned by the CMHC leadership to devote more of his time to the program.

The emergence of the standardized curriculum, the successful provision of services to larger numbers of children, and the stability of the partnership of the three institutions (UMDNJ-CMHC, school system, and Rutgers University Department of Psychology) are described in detail elsewhere (Elias & Clabby, 1984; Elias & Clabby, in press, b). In our effort to look for benchmarks toward institutionalization, a decision of great relevance appears to be the decision made by the three institutions to take on an action-research approach to the longitudinal study of the acquisition, use and impact of social problem solving skills in children's lives and the technology for delivering school-based competence-enhancement and preventive services in this domain.

As Commins (1986) notes, the completion of Stage I towards institutionalization is marked by the host organization's decision to support its continuation. In order to be reasonably sure of their investment, potential external action-research funding sponsors, such as government agencies and private foundations, expect a formal commitment that the involved institutions can and are willing to play a formal multi-year part in supporting and nourishing the project.

To this end, therefore, letters of long-term support for the Social Problem Solving Program were written by significant institutional leaders for the UMDNJ-CMHC at Piscataway, Rutgers University, and the host school system. Completion of Stage I was marked by these institutions offering their commitment to a long-term relationship, a commitment that in our case was sealed by the awarding of substantial, multi-year, action-research funding support first by the William T. Grant Foundation and then by the National Institute of Mental Health.

STAGE TWO: IMPLEMENTATION AND EXPANSION OF THE INNOVATION

Once the commitment for a long-term effort is secured, progress toward true institutionalization is marked by an ongoing action-research feedback and program renewal system where implementors make informed service delivery adjustments in a continued, visable, and persistent effort toward fit with the sponsoring institutions.

In the school-based social problem solving program, the ongoing action-research cycle is two-tiered, in that the cycle continues at the initial grade level at which the program was first carried out (fourth grade), and also continues longitudinally, as cohorts of students move through succeeding grades. In the case of the ISA-SPS Program, the information continued to be obtained concerning the strength, breadth, and duration of effects, and this, of course, impacted upon subsequent program scope and design.

For successful completion of Stage Two, a program must go beyond being seen as a staff member's "project"; it must receive formal and explicit recognition as a *CMHC* program. In the present case, the ISA-SPS Program gradually became viewed as a formal consultation and education program of an outpatient clinic of the CMHC. Its purview was expanded to include other schools in the outpatient unit's catchment area. The ISA-SPS Program continued in this status for three years. During this time, the program leadership was setting into motion processes that led to the successful completion of Stage Two and movement into Stage Three. Specifically, (a) the program focus expanded to be able to be in compliance with local and statewide educational mandates (e.g., for family life education, substance abuse prevention); (b) results of the program were compiled and visibly disseminated locally, statewide, and nationally through reports, publications, and presentations; (c) networking with an increasing array of service providers, service consumers, policy makers, child advocates, and staff from child-serving agencies led the program to be better known and generated an increased demand for program services; and (d) there was continuity on both the core mission of the program and its central leadership, thus affording the program with the revered status of being like "your old, comfortable pair of shoes"—a source of reliability, stability, and perceived positive quality in a wider world in flux.

STAGE THREE: INSTITUTIONALIZATION OF AN INNOVATION AS AN ACCEPTED ORGANIZATIONAL ENTITY

Movement of the ISA-SPS Program into Stage Three—which Commins (1986) described as a point at which a program is routinized as a part of the central functioning of an agency or organization—was propelled by the receipt of a grant from the Middlesex County (NJ) Mental Health Administration and County Freeholders (government) to set up social problem solving programs in two large municipalities outside the traditional catchment area of the CMHC. Again, the grant necessitated that the CMHC make commitments of in-kind and other supportive resources and that the co-director of the program from UMDNJ-CMHC be given the status to negotiate affiliative arrangements with the county, the municipalities' school districts, and other CMHCs which served those schools.

Heretofore, funding had centered on support for the research base of the program; however, the following research findings provided evidence that a promising service technology could be developed from the work done to date: children trained in social problem solving skills demonstrated, when compared to controls (a) more sensitivity to others' feelings, (b) greater understanding of behavioral consequences, (c) increased ability to size up interpersonal situations and plan appropriate action, and (d) higher self-esteem. Further, they were seen by their teachers as better adjusted, were sought out by their peers for help with problems, handled the difficult transition to middle school with less stress, and were using what they learned in social problem solving lessons in situations outside of the classroom. The new support was targeted toward developing a county-wide dissemination capacity, known as the Middlesex County (NJ) Social Problem Solving (SPS) Training Unit. Its mission, as set by the county government, was to bring SPS technology to schools within the catchment areas of two other CMHCs in the county.

With this start-up money, two very large and highly visible school districts became involved in developing SPS programs.

Training procedures were further developed, refined, and took on an increasingly sophisticated look, e.g., various training videotapes were produced.

The modest funding for the new SPS Training Unit continued to flow yearly from the county government. The continual dissemination of outcome studies, yearly increases in the numbers of county children serviced, the publication of an award-winning book by the co-directors (Clabby & Elias, 1986), and the enthusiasm of the teachers and administrators worked to continue to generate interest in the project. More of the involved school districts began to pay for SPS consultation services through grants they had written or from their own local budgets.

Within the sponsoring CMHC, other benchmarks towards institutionalization about which Yin (1979) and Commins (1986) have written were also being reached. In the original hosting public school system, SPS had begun as an add-on or extra program and then began to influence the primary mission of the school system, which was academic skill acquisition. This was marked by such features as the development in the schools of SPS book reports in language arts, and using SPS as a way to teach library research skills. So too, this initially small consultation and education project began to influence the primary mission of its sponsoring CMHC. For example, a comprehensive youth suicide prevention project was developing at the CMHC and among its initial service components were lessons for adolescents which adopted the social problem solving approach as a way to show young people that they can be empowered with a coping skill to combat this critical problem. The suicide prevention program gained large statewide recognition and allowed the SPS approach to become better known not only to the external community but also to key staff within the sponsoring CMHC.

Additionally, for several years the ISA-SPS Project had begun to successfully work in the schools with significantly troubled students who were classified educationally as emotionally disturbed. Clinicians in the CMHC began to use SPS techniques, forged in a prevention context, to help in their remediative work with clients. For example, a clinical group for emotionally disturbed children in the CMHC's Child Day Hospital was begun and led by SPS and Child

Day Hospital staff. This adaptation of SPS technology also filtered into the work done with adult clients. Specifically, components of the SPS approach were adapted by a CMHC clinician, trained by SPS staff, for use with a group of adult aftercare clients at the CMHC's clinic in the inner city. In a gradual way, the learnings of what was once a small consultation and education project, originally given sanction to better the relationship between the CMHC and a local school system, were now influencing some of the primary and core functions of the CMHC.

The most significant milestone toward institutionalization has been the announcement by the University of Medicine and Dentistry of New Jersey that its Community Mental Health Center at Piscataway had created a Social Problem Solving Unit, on an organizational par with the other service delivery units of the CMHC. The program staff's salaries shifted to "hard lines" and the CMHC psychologist responsible for the program was promoted to become the director of the new unit and Chief Psychologist for the UMDNJ-CMHC at Piscataway on a reporting and accountability line on a par with the directors of the other service delivery units, e.g., adult hospital, psychiatric emergency service, among others.

There are other more recent developments that validate and solidify the various institutions' initial decisions to commit to the project. Of particular interest to the UMDNJ-CMHC and Rutgers University constituency was the announcement that the program was named the recipient of the Lela Rowland Prevention Award by the National Mental Health Association (NMHA) as an outstanding example of effective prevention programming and the accompanying commitment by the NMHA to help disseminate the program nationwide. In addition, the Social Problem Solving Unit has been cited as a model program by the U.S. Department of Justice's Office of Juvenile Justice and Delinquency Prevention. Of particular validation to the school systems was the news that the program was selected by the New Jersey Department of Education as one of three model prevention programs in the State. As part of this designation, the Social Problem Solving Program became part of a State Department of Education grant program whereby school districts could secure funds from the State to contract for prevention services from the Social Problem Solving Program.

In becoming a bona fide and permanent service delivery unit of the CMHC, the SPS Unit now has a mission to bring quality SPS programming to as many children as possible. This move of institutionalizing the SPS Unit by a major state medical university may be a unique practice development in the country and assures the longevity needed to be able to provide a solid, visible base for competence enhancement and prevention services over the long term. The history of the development of the SPS Unit is an important example of how consultation and education services might evolve. Occurrences such as the growth and development of the Social Problem Solving Program are indications that some CMHC administrations do have a genuine interest in and commitment to the mental *health* of the community. There can be no more tangible signs of that commitment than the budget lines, space, and support resources given by the UMDNJ-CMHC to the SPS Unit. Competence enhancement and prevention are indeed alive and well in CMHCs and are viable and necessary foci in an upcoming era of more carefully scrutinized health and mental health care.

REFERENCES

Allen, G.J., & Associates. (1976). *Community psychology and the schools: A behaviorally-oriented multilevel prevention approach*. Hillsdale, NJ: Erlbaum.

Clabby, J.F., & Elias, M.J. (1986). *Teach your child decision making*. New York: Doubleday.

Commins, W.W. (1986). *Institutionalization of mental health innovations in the schools*. Doctoral dissertation, Graduate School of Applied and Professional Psychology, Rutgers University, New Brunswick, NJ.

Elardo, P., & Cooper, B. (1977). *AWARE: Activities for social development*. Reading, MA: Addison-Wesley.

Elias, M.J., & Clabby, J.F. (1984). Integrating social and affective education into public school curriculum and instruction. In C. Maher, R. Illbach, & J. Zims (Eds.), *Organizational psychology in the schools: A handbook for professionals* (pp. 143-172). Springfield, IL: C.C. Thomas.

Elias, M.J. (1985). *Formative and summative evaluation of the Improving Social Awareness-Social Problem Solving Primary Prevention Curriculum Program*. New Brunswick, NJ: Rutgers University.

Elias, M.J., & Clabby, J.F. (in press, a). *Social skills and social decision making for the elementary grades: Curriculum and group activities*. Rockville, MD: Aspen.

Elias, M.J., & Clabby, J.F. (in press, b). *Building children's problem solving and decision-making skills: A school-based approach to prevention and remediation*. San Francisco: Jossey-Bass.

Elias, M.J., & Maher, C. (1983). Social and affective development of children: A programmatic perspective. *Exceptional Children*, *49*, 339-348.

Kendall, P., & Hollon, S. (1979). *Cognitive-behavioral intervention: Theory, research and procedures*. New York: Academic Press.

Masterpasqua, F. (1981). Toward a synergism of development and community psychology. *American Psychologist*, *36*, 782-786.

Rutter, M. (1980). *Changing youth in a changing society*. Cambridge, MA: Harvard University Press.

Spivack, G., Platt, J., & Shure, M. (1976). *The problem solving approach to adjustment*. San Francisco: Jossey-Bass.

Yin, R. (1979). *Changing urban bureaucracies: How new practices become routinized*. Lexington, MA: Lexington Books.

The Development and Management of Prevention Services Within a Comprehensive, Medical School-Based, Community Mental Health Center

Steven W. Godin
Lucille Carr-Kaffashan
Paulette Moore Hines
Community Mental Health Center at Piscataway
University of Medicine and Dentistry of New Jersey

SUMMARY. Little has been written about the development and management of prevention services within applied settings. In this paper, the authors (1) present a historical overview and theoretical considerations relevant to prevention work, (2) describe the specific evolution of prevention services within a medical school-based community mental health center, and (3) summarize the array of prevention services offered within this center. It is hoped that this paper will serve as a useful guide for those involved in the planning and delivery of prevention activities.

Authors' note: "It is with sincere appreciation that we wish to acknowledge Mr. Gary Lamson, UMDNJ's Vice President for Mental Health Services. His vision and support have been critical to the development of our center's prevention services. In addition, his help was invaluable in our efforts to reconstruct the historical perspective which is presented in this article. We also wish to acknowledge the many dedicated staff members of our center. Without their creativity and willingness to go above and beyond the call of duty, there would be no prevention program for us to describe."

Reprints may be obtained from Steven Godin, Office of Prevention Services, Community Mental Health Center, University of Medicine and Dentistry of New Jersey, Piscataway, NJ 08854.

This article presents a description of an exemplary prevention program run through the "Office of Prevention Services" located within the Community Mental Health Center of the University of Medicine and Dentistry of New Jersey. In our description, we will first address what we perceive to be the key management and organizational activities necessary for the development and maintenance of hearty, efficacious prevention programs. The second section of the paper will outline the history of the center's prevention services and the application of certain theoretical notions to the various developmental phases of the program's growth. In the last section, we will provide a summary of the current prevention services offered within our center. The various services are categorized using John Morgan's (in press) typology system. Inasmuch as the history of prevention services in our mental health center has corresponded to the history of the consultation and education movement, we will begin the article with a brief discussion of the latter.

HISTORICAL AND THEORETICAL CONSIDERATIONS

The consultation and education (C&E) movement received its impetus in 1963 when Congress passed Public Law 88-164 which provided funding for a national network of community mental health centers. This legislation required all federally funded centers to provide consultation and education services to promote mental health and prevent mental illness in the local community. In 1975, amendments to this legislation established special categorical funding support allowing for the expansion of consultation and education programs. These amendments recommended that each federally funded community mental health center employ at least one full-time staff member to be responsible for consultation and education activities.

Despite federal funding efforts, community mental health centers allocated an average of only 5% of their total funding to consultation and education programs. The majority of funding was directed toward providing clinical and rehabilitation services (Snow & Newton, 1976). By 1981, the Omnibus Budget Reconcilitation Act (Public Law 97-35) brought a basic change in the federal philosophy, role, and funding of community mental health center services.

This legislation led to the implementation of the ADM block grant program which eliminated special categorical support for consultation and education (Bevilacqua, 1982; Brown, 1983).

As a result of these shifts in funding, substantial modifications occurred in the 1980s in the provision of consultation and education services within federally funded community mental health centers. A study conducted by Backer and Levine (1983) cited that 79% of the community mental health centers surveyed reported shifts in their consultation and education programs as a result of this change in funding. A little over half (53%) of the centers reported specific cutbacks in C&E staff and program activities.

While funding cutbacks have been attributed to be the major cause for the decline in C&E service delivery, there are many community mental health centers that continue to successfully engage in consultation and education activities (Backer & Levine, 1983). There appear to be other important mediating factors that determine whether or not C&E services will survive, and perhaps flourish, in an agency. Specifically, some have suggested the importance of organizational activity and ideologies of key staff members that create an environment conducive to C&E program development (see Broskowski & Baker, 1974; Cherniss, 1977; Ketterer & Perkins, 1977; Perlmutter & Silverman, 1973; Snow & Newton, 1976).

Until recently, most of the consultation and education program development literature has focused primarily upon the qualities of, and the strategies for working with, the "consultee" or target population. Little attention has been given to the qualities and circumstances relevant to the social milieu of the larger organization and the dynamic exchange that exists between staff members and this social milieu. Too often, prevention practitioners have failed to keep in the forefront of their planning the notion that the success of consultation and education efforts is highly operator-dependent (see Rossi, 1978). While assessment of the target population is vital, assessment and intervention must also be conducted within the consultant's own organization to facilitate successful program development and management of consultation and education.

Recently, Trickett, Kelly, and Vincent (1985) have addressed the importance of understanding the interaction and interdependence that exists between the program developer and his/her organization. Incorporating an "ecological perspective," Trickett and his colleagues have illustrated a set of principles useful in guiding the prevention program coordinator toward effective systems consultation and program development. This paper serves to expand the ecological framework and to illustrate the application of ecological theory within four phases of development that have occurred since the inception of our center's prevention program. The four phases of program development include: (1) Assessment of the Organizational Environment; (2) Program Planning and Implementation; (3) Program Maintenance and Evaluation; and (4) Program Consolidation.

Assessment of the Organizational Environment

A central diagnostic task in both consultation and program development is first to identify, assess, and if necessary, attempt to redistribute organizational resources. Resources can be any phenomena or entities that serve to enhance the successful functioning of the organization. Examples of resources could be individuals, relationships, departments within the organization, and particular events that have occurred in the organization's history. Raber (1984) suggests that the key prerequisites for successful prevention programming are a positive organizational history and a center director who values consultation and education services. Without administrative backing, even the most creative, efficient programming can fail (see Cherniss, 1977). If these organizational conditions do not exist, the program planner's energy is better spent manipulating organizational resources (conducting primary prevention) in a way to assure the necessary support. Once administrative backing is achieved, the program developer can attempt to create and/or activate key organizational resources to facilitate prevention program development. Raber (1984) suggests a strategic planning approach that assesses the organization's constituencies, range of services, internal relationships of staff, finances, facilities, staff development, and training.

In the initial planning stages, the program developer may wish to make use of planned change models such as "A-VICTORY" (see Davis, 1973; Davis & Salasin, 1980). A-VICTORY is an acronym for eight dimensions one may assess to determine the organization's readiness for change or innovation. The *A* dimension is an assessment of the organization's *Ability*. The program developer needs to determine whether the organization has the necessary capabilities and resources to implement and maintain a prevention program. The *V* dimension is an assessment of the organization's *Values*. One must determine whether the values inherent in the organization are congruent with the ideology of preventive intervention. The *I* dimension is an assessment of the organization's awareness of relevant *Information*. That is, one must assess whether current staff have sufficient expertise in the delivery of preventive interventions. The *C* dimension is an assessment of *Circumstances* or environmental factors which may affect program development. These include assessing specific organizational factors which could potentially interfere with the successful development of the prevention program. The *T* dimension is an assessment of *Timing*. The program developer needs to determine the most appropriate time to implement the prevention program. The *O* dimension is an assessment of the level of *Obligation* the administration has toward the delivery of prevention services. The *R* dimension is an assessment of potential *Resistance* that key staff may have toward prevention program development prior to implementation. The final dimension *Y* is the assessment of intended *Yield*. The program developer needs to anticipate the potential benefits and costs of the program being considered and to hypothesize whether a particular intervention will have a positive impact on the organization as a whole, thus creating a greater likelihood for future administrative support.

Program Planning and Implementation

Given the organizational conditions which exist in a particular mental health center, the next task of the program developer is to select/design the type of program that will have a high probability of success. After comprehensive assessment and manipulation of organizational resources and variables, the program developer can anticipate successful implementation of the program.

Particular attention needs to be given to the incentive structures within the organization, as well as the target population's need. Depending on the incentives within a given center, prevention programming may be seen as more valuable by the administration if it first concentrates on developing innovative, resource generating programs such as employee assistance programs, consultation to health maintenance organizations, organizational wellness programs, and so forth (see Backer & Levine, 1983; Erchul & Backer, 1984; Raber, 1984). Another approach to increase the value of prevention programming is for the program developer to focus on developing interventions that enhance center visibility in the community. Prevention programs that address the current "hot issues" such as alcohol abuse prevention, drunk driving prevention, adolescent pregnancy prevention, and teenage suicide prevention may serve to increase the credibility and visibility of the center in the community and professional field. Successful, resource generating programs create a resource-rich ecosystem within the organization which may increase support for the development of important programs that cannot be self-supporting. Resources from high resource generating prevention programs may be allowed to trickle down to low resource generating programs. Prevention programs that are nonrevenue or low resource generating thus become interdependent on resource generating programs. This recycling of resources approach (see Trickett et al., 1985) is essentially a "republican model" of providing prevention services.

Throughout the program planning and implementation phase, it is essential that the program developer keep the agency director aware of program progress. In addition, providing information throughout the organization about recent developments can help staff to assimilate and accommodate the ideology and values of prevention work. Finally, the program developer needs to be proactive rather than reactive in creating an organizational environment which will facilitate the healthy development of the prevention program. Sensitivity to sudden changes in organizational environment and/or access to resources is essential. Davis' (1973) A-VICTORY planned change model can be a useful tool in assessing organizational readiness throughout the planning and implementation phase.

Program Maintenance and Evaluation

Once the program developer has a prevention program underway, efforts should center around daily maintenance and periodic evaluation. Inadequate maintenance is likely to result in program dysfunction or possible program breakdown. Anticipating possible obstacles to program growth and developing contingency plans are essential. Continuous monitoring and allocation of current and future resources is also necessary to insure program strength and growth. One type of resource is those individuals who are capable of assuming responsibility for the future maintenance and care of given intervention(s). Prevention staff duties are defined as each staff member understands his or her role in the maintenance of the program.

In an agency that is resource rich, that values preventive efforts, or that has adequately trained staff, programming may be implemented under a specialist model (see Bergner, 1981; Raber, 1984). In the specialist model, all prevention efforts are carried out by full-time prevention specialists who devote all their work efforts towards prevention activities. One drawback of this model is the possibility of isolation from direct service staff. This isolation enhances the possibility of staff misunderstandings and devaluing of each other's roles in the combined efforts of the mental health center. These misunderstandings can create organizational resistance toward preventive interventions and, if strong enough, may eventually undermine future preventive efforts. Furthermore, if preventive efforts are contingent on "soft funding" (i.e., grants, local funding, etc.), an alternative model may be more appropriate. Expiration of soft funding can create high risk for program or staff termination.

In agencies where resources are limited, or where key staff have a tendency to lean toward a more clinical ideology, a generalist model of administration is recommended (see Bergner, 1981; Raber, 1984). In this model, preventive efforts are carried out as part of the staff's overall duties. This model is recommended for small agencies that are unable to afford specialized staff. The generalist model is also a valuable approach in those agencies which have staff who are unfamiliar with or place less value on prevention. Staff with clinical roles or ideologies are more likely to come into contact with fellow staff who are conducting prevention activities and to develop an understanding and acceptance of the prevention service element. Furthermore, the generalist model affords opportunities for staff to gain experience and develop a knowledge-base in conducting prevention activities. Many mental health professionals have never received training in prevention work; others know how, but do not label their work as prevention. One of the drawbacks of this model is that generalists are at high risk for role ambiguity and role stress. For agencies that have heavy clinical demands, staff members often experience internal or external pressure to provide direct service while prevention becomes a second priority. Furthermore, the "mind set" to conduct prevention versus clinical services is likely to be very different. Generalists need to adopt a flexible cognitive style so that they can quickly access the various skills and strategies needed to function successfully in both roles.

Program developers may also use a mixed model of implementation (see Raber, 1984). In this model, one or more staff members are involved in prevention services full-time, while other staff devote a certain percentage of their work toward prevention efforts. This model has all the positive and negative qualities of the specialist and generalist models. Usually, this model is used only in very large organizations or agencies with ample resources.

Record keeping to document how resources are allocated and generated is vital in the management of prevention activities (Raber, 1984). Routine qualitative and quantitative evaluation of various preventive interventions is necessary to assess the utility of the prevention program. Based on program evaluation feedback, program developers can decide which interventions may require greater access to resources and which services are a resource liability in the ecosystem. Using an action-research methodology in program evaluation and proper record keeping, the program developer can mediate the succession (evolution or the assimilation and accommodation of the ecosystem) of the prevention program (Price, 1980; Raber, 1984; Stanford, 1970; Trickett et al., 1985). Based on evaluation results, the program developer can determine which intervention methods are efficacious and which methods need revision. Methodological design in one preventive intervention may prove to be useful in the design of another intervention. This cross-pollination leads to the creation of hybrid programs.

As prevention technology advances, so too must the knowledge base of the staff connected to prevention services. Staff development in theories of prevention, preventive interventions, theories of groups/systems, organizational theory and development, consultation theory, and research and program evaluation methods is essential in the ongoing maintenance of the prevention program (Raber, 1984). Students and faculty from social science departments within local universities often can provide students to assist in conducting daily interventions and/or the technical assistance needed to conduct ongoing evaluations of existing preventive interventions.

Program Consolidation

Some interventions will be assets in resource generation, while others will be liabilities. Interventions which generate significant resources should receive significant staff attention and energy. Difficult decisions will need to be made as to how many low resource-generating preventive interventions can be in existence at any given time. In addition, certain programs may become so successful that significant staff energy may be needed to manage the program's growth. Often, successful programs can become so large that they begin to be at risk for failure due to poor management or the inability to conduct adequate evaluation. It is at this point that an organization may wish to move toward consolidation and re-allocation of resources. During the consolidation process, the program developer will be involved in activities similar to those of the program planning and implementation stage.

HISTORY AND PHASES OF DEVELOPMENT OF PREVENTION SERVICES, UMDNJ – COMMUNITY MENTAL HEALTH CENTER

In this section, the fifteen year history and development of our mental health center's prevention program will be outlined. For each phase of development, those events and variables critical to the program's growth, continuity, and success will be identified. The overall process is conceptualized within an agricultural metaphor in the hope of concretizing the tasks and considerations which were relevant at each developmental stage (see Table 1 which brings together the center's chronological history, variables considered critical to program continuity and success, theoretical references, and the agricultural metaphor).

In October 1972, the Community Mental Health Center of Rutgers Medical School (as it was then called) opened its doors with a mandate to provide high quality clinical and C&E services to a nine town catchment area in central New Jersey. The population to be served was, and continues to be, widely divergent, encompassing the urban poor, a university community of students and faculty, and both blue collar and upper middle class families.

The first developmental phase of the center's C&E program (Assessment of the Organizational Environment) can be likened to the process by which a farmer assesses the growing environment, selects plants, and gathers nutrients (see Table 1, Phase 1). The sociopolitical climate was one which valued social activism and encouraged the development of non-traditional, community-oriented mental health programs. Federal funding was specifically earmarked for C&E programs, and the center opened with a distinct, and well-fertilized, centralized C&E unit called the Community Systems Service (CSS). Given its emphasis on needs assessment, community organizing, and advocacy, CSS played a significant role in establishing data which was used to plan and develop all the center's program elements. This role was recognized and valued by the center's first executive director, who consequently allowed the unit considerable flexibility and protection from the demands of clinical services. Just as seeds germinate best in loose soil, protected from harsh weather, so too CSS flourished under these conditions. In addition, the center's planning committee initiated a recruitment process which favored the selection of "community minded" staff for clinical units, thereby creating an organizational climate of commitment to community involvement and interventions. Community-minded clinical staff are not unlike the hybrid seeds and plants chosen for their ability to withstand changing and unpredictable environmental conditions.

Table 1

Phases of Development

Phase I. Assessment of the Organizational Environment

Year	Key Events	Critical Variables	Ecological/Management Theory Contributions	Agricultural Metaphor
1971	CMHC Planning Committee convened	1. Goal of CMHC director to establish CMHC identity and reputation in the community	1. Program developer's relationship to the CMHC director (Raber, 1984)	1. Fertile & protected environment
1972	In October, CMHC opens with independent, centralized C&E unit, called the Community Systems Service (CSS)	2. Socio-political climate which valued social activism & "community mental health," and a mandate to provide C&E services	2. Assessment and activation of resources (Trickett, Kelly, & Vincent, 1985)	2. Fertile & supportive environment
1973	Federal CMHC funding grant received			
		3. Independent C&E unit, isolated from clinical services, with flexible internal organization of unit	3. Facilitative organizational structure; specialist model (Raber, 1984)	3. Planting site-choice of a loose (flexible) planting medium, protected site
		4. Selection of "community minded" staff for clinical units, community organizing specialists for C&E unit	4. Strategic planning (Raber, 1984)	4. Selection of hybrid seeds and plants
		5. Specific funding for C&E (federal grant)	5. Assessment of CMHC readiness through A-Victory model (Davis, 1973)	5. Adequate nutrients and water

During the early part of the program planning and implementation phase (Phase II), the newly germinated C&E program was nurtured and protected so that the "seedling" could reach its full strength and potency (see Table 1, Phase II-A). A new center director who was more actively supportive of C&E, given his background and values, took over during this period. In addition, an amendment to the Federal Community Mental Health Centers Act in 1975 expanded funding for C&E services and thus ensured that adequate "nutrients" would be available to continue to feed the growing C&E program.

At the same time that CSS was at the height of its operation, alternate planting sites were being readied to accomodate the further expansion of C&E services. Just as seedlings are often transplanted to maximize their growth and reduce competition for resources, so too were the center's C&E services transplanted.

At the point when three outpatient satellite units were located out of the main center building, each with specific communities (or sub-catchment area) for which it was responsible, C&E Coordinator and Educator-Clinician roles were established in each unit. Educator-Clinicians were mental health professionals designated to serve as liaisons with the local school system in a given community. These changes clearly laid the groundwork for a decentralized, community-based model of C&E service delivery which would allow for program expansion; program flexibility, in that services could be designed to meet specific community needs; and program protection, in that these units could be more adaptive to fluctuating environmental conditions which might alternately favor clinical or C&E service elements.

In the latter part of Phase II (see Table 1, Phase II-B) the transplanting of the C&E program was fully implemented. The centralized C&E unit (CSS) was dissolved and its staff re-assigned. Two projects which were developed by CSS grew so big that they required their own separate plots of land, and thus were spun off into distinct units of the mental health center. Both have grown substantially and continue to operate at this writing.

The New Brunswick Outreach Unit remains the closest in philosophy and operation to the original CSS unit. Its mission is to foster the health and empowerment of the urban poor and minority popu-

TABLE 1 (continued)

Phase II. Program Planning and Implementation

Key Events	Critical Variables	Ecological/Management Theory Contributions	Agricultural Metaphor
A. 1974-1976 -Centralized C&E unit (CSS) with approximately one dozen staff	1. New CMHC director is more actively supportive of CSS and the mission of C&E	1. Program developer's relationship to the Center Director (Raber, 1984)	1. Supportive and protected enrironment
-Three outpatient units are moved out of main Center building to increase accessibility to the community	2. Amendment to CMHC act in 1975 which expanded funding for C&E programming and re-affirmed value of C&E services	2. Assessment of CMHC readiness through A-Victory model (Davis, 1973)	2. Adequate nutrients & water
Educator-clinician (school liaison) and C&E coordinator roles are established on each unit	3. Connections to the 9 catchment area communities are more firmly established	3. Recycling of resources; adaptation; and interdependence within the ecosystem (Trickett, Kelly, & Vincent, 1985)	3. Preparing alternate planting sites

TABLE 1 (continued)

Key Events	Critical Variables	Ecological/Management Theory Contributions	Agricultural Metaphor
B. 1977-1978 -Current CMHC director takes over -Centralized C&E unit (CSS) is dissolved & staff re-assigned; two CSS projects with distinct identities become separate units of the CMHC (New Brunswick Outreach and Community Outreach Program for Senior Adults -Outpatient units are designated as blended clinical and C&E units	1. New CMHC director has a community organizing background, was on original CMHC planning committee, and was a staff member of CSS	1. Program developer's relationship to the Center Director (Raber, 1984)	1. A master farmer with a feel for the land
	2. Decentralization of C&E service delivery	2. Facilitative organizational structure; generalist model (Raber, 1984)	2. Transplanting to more fertile sites, with more space for growth
	3. In light of national trend toward more traditional clinical interventions, and in anticipation of end of federal grant in 1980, community and clinical interventions are blended, and an emphasis is placed on income generating projects and on better accountability for the extent and value of C&E services delivered	3. Strategic planning (Raber, 1984) Republican model of C&E program development (Backer & Levine, 1985; Erchul & Backer, 1984)	3. Transplanting to a more protected site, introduction of new hybrid plants, and closer monitoring of plant production

lations of New Brunswick through community advocacy, organizing, and educational activities.

COPSA (formerly the Community Outreach Program for Senior Adults, now known as the Comprehensive Services for the Aging Unit) was also established at that time to provide outreach and advocacy services for senior citizens throughout the catchment area. All other C&E services were essentially transplanted to the three outpatient units, and each blended unit became responsible for implementing both clinical and C&E services for its sub-catchment area communities. Given the national trend at the time toward more traditional clinical interventions, and the anticipated end of the center's federal funding grant in 1980, it is clear that the blending of clinical and community interventions played a critical role in safeguarding the center's C&E program. The decentralized model allowed for greater flexibility and adaptability, and much less vulnerability at the point when specific C&E funding was eliminated. At any given time, approximately two-thirds of all "clinical" staff were engaged in C&E work at some level.

The other highly significant variable during this developmental phase was the designation of a new center director. This individual, who is also the current Director and Vice-President for Mental Health Services for UMDNJ, holds a graduate degree in community organizing, was on the original mental health center planning committee, and was a staff member of CSS. His background, therefore, combined a commitment to and understanding of community level interventions with a thorough knowledge of the center and the catchment area it serves. Throughout all other phases of development, and up through the present time, his vision, support, and guidance have been critical to the success of the center's C&E program.

The early part of the Program Maintenance and Evaluation phase (Phase III) was a period of moderate program growth, with considerable emphasis placed on the development of an effective system for managing the center's C&E program (see Table 1, Phase III-A). While the decentralized model ensured program continuity and scope, it also created the need for more systematic service coordination, record-keeping, and communication procedures. Growing plants can become unwieldy if a systematic pattern of maintenance

TABLE 1 (continued)

Phase III. Program Maintenance and Evaluation

	Key Events	Critical Variables	Ecological/Management Theory Contributions	Agricultural Metaphor
A. 1978-1982	Emphasis is placed on the management of C&E; service coordination, record-keeping and communication procedures are designed. In 1978, annual centerwide C&E reports are instituted, and in 1981, a center C&E manual which delineates philosophies and procedures is distributed. In 1980, a centerwide C&E coordinator is designated	1. Increasing financial concerns coupled with increasing demands for service necessitate more careful management and planning. Staff are encouraged to seek grants and fees for service	1. Strategic planning (Raber, 1984)	1. Preparation for drought conditions; water conservation plus the development of new irrigation systems
		2. High quality C&E services are seen as a marketing tool for the center as a whole; as such, careful documentation is emphasized as well as statewide and national promotion of C&E activities	2. Strategic planning Record keeping (Raber, 1984)	2. Harvesting the fruit and, after careful weighing and measuring, taking it to market

	Key Events	Critical Variables	Ecological/Management Theory Contributions	Agricultural Metaphor
B. 1983-1986	-Three outpatient unit C&E coordinators share the role of Centerwide C&E Coordinator, and function as a C&E management team -Staff from various CMHC units are pulled together to develop centerwide C&E projects -Funding crisis threatens both clinical and C&E programs	1. Funding crisis, increased demand for both C&E and clinical services, and increased pressure for accountability and paperwork from reviewing agencies (e.g., JCAH, State Division of Mental Health and Hospitals)	1. A-Victory model (Davis, 1973)	1. Threat of drought and total depletion of resources
		2. Generation of grant money and fees for service	2. Recycling of resources (Tricket, Kelly, & Vincent, 1985)	2. Replenishing the soil
		3. Pooling of resources; reduction of smaller projects; and increased emphasis on multifaceted, comprehensive projects with evaluation components	3. Recycling of resources (Trickett, Kelly, & Vincent, 1985) Republican model (Backer & Levine, 1985; Erchul & Backer, 1984)	3. Pruning and plant thinning so as to concentrate resources on the most productive plants
		4. Careful attention to those mental health topic areas which are of particular social/political relevance in the community	4. Strategic planning (Raber, 1984) Recycling of resources (Trickett, Kelly & Vincent, 1985)	4. Continuing assessment of soil and environmental conditions which would support or threaten the plants
		5. Staff development, via inservice training and interchange, as well as participation in local/national organizations and conferences	5. Action-research program evaluation (Price, 1980; Sanford, 1970) Mixed model (Raber, 1984)	5. Cross-pollination to ensure adequate production levels and to develop new products

is not instituted. During this phase, a system for documenting staff time spent on C&E activities was developed, annual centerwide C&E reports which catalogued all C&E activities in a given year were instituted, a C&E manual was written, and a centerwide C&E coordinator (who also functioned as a C&E coordinator for one of the outpatient units) was designated.

The improved documentation of C&E services was related to program success and continuity for two reasons. First, the socio-political climate was one of increased demand for accountability and financial belt-tightening. Thus, it was important to demonstrate program productivity and the appropriate utilization of staff, as well as involvement with target populations and problems which were considered high priority by funding sources. This is not unlike the process by which a farmer must predict crop yields in order to secure financing. Second, the documentation and publicizing of high quality, enduring C&E projects (both statewide and nationally) was extremely useful in promoting and marketing the center as a whole, insofar as visibility and credibility were enhanced. This latter effect is, of course, also related to funding, although in a more indirect, generalized manner.

Increased financial concerns during this phase also necessitated more careful management and allocation of resources, and thus a process of pruning and replenishing the soil was begun. In preparation for funding cuts and the end of the federal grant in 1980, staff were encouraged to aggressively seek grants and fees for service. This represented a significant shift, insofar as nearly all C&E services had previously been offered free of charge to the community. As such, a process for training key C&E staff was begun in order to help them feel more comfortable about, and more skilled in, negotiating fees for services and in developing grant proposals.

During the latter part of Phase III (see Table 1, Phase III-B) a number of stressors contributed to a severe strain on existing resources and the experience shared by staff around the center of being stretched to the limit. Some factors which contributed to this stress were a funding crisis which carried with it the threat of layoffs (although fortunately the layoffs were avoided when funding eventually came through), an overwhelming increase in the community's requests for both clinical and C&E services, and increased paperwork and demands for documentation by reviewing agencies. Within this organizational climate, a significant shift occurred when the person serving concurrently as the C&E coordinator for the center and one of the outpatient units left the center. Following this, the three outpatient unit C&E coordinators began to function essentially as a centralized C&E management team. This shift allowed for a more concentrated effort to address the stressors mentioned above, and in so doing, laid the groundwork for another growth spurt for the center's C&E program.

The C&E management team mobilized a number of strategies to conserve resources and to reduce the stress of the existing harsh environmental conditions:

1. Administrative support and encouragement were offered to staff in their quest for grant money and fees for service. C&E revenues increased significantly during these years, which served to replenish the soil from which the C&E program had grown.
2. Many smaller, short-term, or single session C&E projects were pruned out, and staff were encouraged to collaborate on multifaceted, enduring C&E projects with evaluation components.
3. A pooling of resources was facilitated by bringing together staff from various units across the center to develop centerwide C&E projects. The goals were to increase efficiency by avoiding duplication of efforts, to reach a wider audience in the community, to enhance staff development and support, and to develop new products through a cross-pollination of existing products. This was the initial step back toward a more centralized model of service delivery.
4. Careful attention was given to the development of staff specialists in all mental health topic areas which were of particular social and/or political relevance in the community, including suicide, AIDS, sexual abuse and incest, latchkey children, drug abuse, alzheimer's disease, and so forth.

As is often the case, however, measures which are implemented to address one set of problems can generate a new set of even thornier ones. Paradoxically, key C&E staff became victims of their own success in that the strategies outlined above facilitated the development of more comprehensive, income-producing projects which required more and more staff time. Given the decentralized, mixed model of service delivery which had been adopted years earlier, key C&E staff (i.e., C&E Coordinators from various units, Educator-Clinicians, and a few special project staff, whose job descriptions included at least 50% time for C&E) were experiencing severe role strain in trying to balance the delivery of both C&E and clinical services. In addition, staff who were responsible for coordinating the delivery of clinical services expressed increasing frustration at the staff time that was gradually, but surely, being diverted from clinical to C&E services. To further complicate matters, the initiation of a major expansion in a number of program elements of the center other than C&E (e.g., the doubling of inpatient beds for children and adolescents) contributed as well to a significant drain on existing resources. The addition of new staff lagged behind the expansion of services, and senior staff were engaged in extensive planning activities in addition to their usual program management activities. Clearly, the large number of flourishing, mature plants which had developed at the center were all competing for limited nutrients and space in order to survive.

In order to address these concerns, and to streamline what had become an extremely complex and difficult-to-manage C&E structure, a new strategic planning process was initiated by the center director and the C&E management team. This moved C&E into its fourth developmental phase, consolidation of the program (see Table 1, Phase IV). The major goals for the consolidation were to maximize the utilization of limited resources, to reduce maintenance efforts and costs, and to protect the integrity of both C&E and clinical services. Another goal was to ensure the continuity of the center's major C&E projects, with a particular emphasis on the need to enhance the center's capacity to meaningfully evaluate all such projects. One final goal was to re-organize the program in such a way as to keep step with current trends and philosophies. This involved letting go of the term "C&E" and the development of a centralized Office of Prevention Services with the designation of a full-time project director and full-time staff. The director is respon-

TABLE 1 (continued)

Phase IV. Program Consolidation

	Key Events	Critical Variables	Ecological/Management Theory Contributions	Agricultural Metaphor
1986-1987	-A new strategic planning process for C&E set into motion by the CMHC director and the C&E management team; models for re-organization of C&E program are discussed/evaluated	1. Continued high demand for clinical and C&E services, coupled with CMHC expansion, intensifies the drain on existing resources	1. Recycling of resources; adaptation; interdependence within the eco-system (Trickett, Kelly, Vincent, 1985)	1. Overplanting creates a drain on available nutrients and water, and on caretaking/maintenance capacity
	-Major expansion in a number of program elements of the CMHC (other than C&E)	2. Management concerns regarding excessive and/or inefficient utilization of resources (e.g., staff time) for C&E program and regarding the continuity of major C&E projects necessitate a reorganization of the C&E program	2. The development of enduring prevention programs (Elias, 1985) Recycling of resources (Trickett, et al. 1985) Mixed Model (Raber, 1984)	2. Re-landscaping and re-designation of planting areas so as to maximize resources to reduce maintenance efforts/costs, and to ensure continuity of most productive plants
	-As of summer, 1987 shift toward centralized model of service delivery with the development of an Office of Prevention Services, the reassignment of staff from other units to this office, and the designation of a project director	3. Renewed interest (on national and local levels) in the concepts of prevention, with increased funding opportunities; continued emphasis on evaluation and accountability in relation to funding	3. The development of enduring prevention programs (Elias, 1985) Strategic planning (Raber, 1984)	3. Repackaging of products and improved quality assurance strategies so as to meet demands of current market

sible for coordination of prevention services center-wide. The staff on the unit provide technical assistance to the generalists in the center who implement prevention services. Additionally, the Office of Prevention Services staff are responsible for developing new initiatives, and expanding several preexisting initiatives.

Thus, in its fifteen year history, numerous landscapings of our center's prevention program have resulted in the use of all three models of service delivery in an attempt to keep step with national and local trends and priorities. What follows is a description of the scope and types of prevention services which are currently offered.

OVERVIEW OF CURRENT PREVENTION SERVICES

The University of Medicine and Dentistry of New Jersey Community Mental Health Center at Piscataway presently offers an array of community-based prevention services. Programs span the life cycle, from infants at risk for abuse and/or neglect by their teenaged parents to elderly persons and their families who struggle to cope with the impact of Alzheimer's disease. Our aim has been to be comprehensive with regard to age and developmental levels, major social roles, major geographic areas within our catchment area, major disability areas, and high risk situations within the limitations dictated by staffing and funding resources. Program priorities are based on consideration of the following: (1) guidelines from funding and accrediting agents; (2) demographic data; (3) key informant surveys; (4) community forums; (5) formal needs assessment; (6) the center's organizational plan; (7) staff expertise and time availability; (8) utilization statistics for the CMHC's clinical services; and (9) funding potential.

The issues addressed in any given year may vary but for the most part there is an effort to maintain consistency in focus, as appropriate. The range of issues addressed is broad. A partial listing of issues addressed during the past year includes: separation and divorce; single parenting; parenting skills; stress management; housing, employment, health and empowerment of the urban poor and minorities; suicide prevention, grief resolution and coping skills enhancement for suicide survivors; substance abuse among teens and adults; barriers to healthy functioning for high school dropouts; teen pregnancy and parenting; AIDS; social problem solving among youth and adolescents; latchkey stress among children; the impact of Alzheimer's disease and related disorders on families; urban youth stressors; child abuse and neglect; youth leadership development; support for the caregivers of the mentally ill; gay and lesbian lifestyle stressors; cultural transition stressors; and retirement planning.

Over 63,300 people across the state of New Jersey were direct recipients of the center's prevention services in fiscal year 1987-1988. This figure does not reflect the true number of people impacted as some preventive services do not involve face to face contacts (e.g., media presentations) and thus the people serviced cannot be counted. Over 25,400 hours of prevention-oriented services were provided to the community. Grant funding of $1,090,015 was received in support of six prevention projects. However, the bulk of the remaining services were provided to the recipients at no cost or at reduced cost totaling $130,346 in fee for service revenues. The service hours reported by staff from the various units of the center approximate 14 full-time staff equivalents.

A sample of activities which illustrate the nature of the center's work more specifically is herein offered. The typology of prevention interventions is borrowed fron the work of John Morgan (in press).

General Competency Building

The *Social Problem Solving Project* began in 1979 as a collaboration between the center, a local university, and the public schools. The project targets youth in both regular and special education classes to increase their social competence by equipping them with solid decision making and social problem solving skills. These skills include: (a) the ability to develop detailed and flexible plans to obtain one's goals; (b) the ability to identify problem areas and past feelings and behavioral responses to these problems; (c) knowledge of one's past effectiveness in problem situations; (d) the ability to consider multiple alternatives and strategies in solving problems and predicting potential obstacles; (e) the ability to implement the best alternative or strategies while maintaining sensitivity to others' feelings and perspectives; and (f) the ability to monitor one's experiences in situations and use this information to refine future social problem solving performance. At the present time, the project reaches over 1000 children per year through six program staff and numerous graduate and undergraduate students from Rutgers University who offer intensive training and year-long, on-site consultation to educators. Additional training is provided to parents who have an opportunity to reinforce the skills being taught in the classroom. Several years of evaluation data have been accumulated. The results of numerous evaluations suggest that the model is an effective way of teaching social problem solving skills and that students do practice the skills in their everyday lives.

Specific Coping Skills Training

The *Student Assistance Program* is currently being offered in four high schools and four middle schools. The program goals are to increase awareness about alcohol and drug use, to prevent students from using alcohol and other drugs, and to eliminate alcohol and other drug use among those students who are abusing. Program services include consultation and training with school staff, educational and didactic presentations to classes throughout the year, and individual, group and family sessions and referrals as needed. The program generated $50,000 in revenue from the school districts served while the center assumed the remaining costs for the four staff involved.

In conjunction with a local adult education program, the center administers one of twelve pilot programs in the state for high school dropouts ages 16 to 25. This program, *New Jersey Youth Corps*, strives to provide a second chance for out-of-school and out-of-work young adults to lead satisfying and productive lives. A vital component of the program is assisting enrollees in addressing personal, familial, and interpersonal barriers to success. Specifically, the program offers basic skills instruction, employment readiness instruction, employment survival training, community work experience to establish a work history and references, placement and follow-up services, transportation, and child-care assistance. The center has played a major role in program design at both the local and state levels, particularly in the effort to address attitudinal and socio-personal barriers to success. In addition to individual, group, and family intervention, enrollees participate in personal development and life coping skills workshops. The program has served over 284 adolescents and young adults during the last two years. The program is jointly funded by the New Jersey Division of Adult Education and the New Jersey Department of Community Affairs. Funding for this project over the last three years has exceeded $1,200,000. Evaluation has been limited to outcome variables such as the number of youth earning their diplomas and the number of youth placed in jobs. These results indicate that youth participants in the Youth Corps program have outcome results five times better than those who participate in adult education programs which offer only basic skills instruction. Our project staff are currently completing the design for a demonstration evaluation which will determine what, if any, variables are predictive of program success and examine program impact on various attitudinal and coping skills variables.

Children at Risk: Resources and Interventions, which is better known as CARRI, targets teen parents and their infants. A minimum of 100 teens have been served annually since the program's inception. Six full-time staff offer outreach, support, and guidance to facilitate positive parent-child interactions, teach parenting and infant stimulation skills, promote a positive relationship between teen mothers and their own mothers, encourage responsibility and active involvement of teen fathers, and facilitate coordination of resources for the young parents and their infants. Last year, the program was supported by $244,239 in funds from a federal grant, a private foundation, and block grant funds. Research is underway to examine the impact of program interventions on the level of family and social support as well as resources available to the teens. Program impact on the developmental functioning of the infants is also being assessed.

Community-based educational and skill building programs were also conducted on topics such as living with and caring for the elderly, the mentally ill, and chemically dependent persons. In addition, through the center's *Intoxicated Drivers Project*, 560 persons adjudicated for driving while intoxicated were involved in alcohol education groups. Two six-hour days of educational meetings per month were provided to participants.

Support System Interventions

Phonefriend is a telephone help line for children which was originally established to provide children with support, information and help in solving problems during a time of day when many are at home alone. The program is staffed by a paid coordinator and a group of volunteers trained and supervised through the center. Additionally, there is frequent, behind the scenes consultation, networking, and follow-up with the center and other community agencies to provide services for troubled youngsters.

Phonefriend has received over 15,000 calls during an 18 month period of operation. Although many calls are from children in need of support because of boredom, loneliness, or anxiety, a large percentage of calls are from children asking for help with serious problems, including abuse, neglect, drug and alcohol issues, sexuality issues, peer problems, depression, suicidality, and family problems. Despite the fact that the program was marketed to grammar and middle school children, almost 10% of the calls have come from adolescents. The groundwork is being laid for the addition of a teen line. Information from daily calls is documented and coded for computer analysis. This information about youth concerns and problems has been relayed to parents and others through community symposiums, PTOs, and the like. The information has also proven to be a valuable source of data for youth service planners. Efforts to establish an adequate funding base for the project have been unsuccessful. Thus far, approximately $20,000 has been contributed on an annual basis through a small grant, organizations, and individuals.

Since 1985, a number of staff have been active in collaborating with a community-based foundation on the development and implementation of a system of support for people with AIDS and AIDS related complex and their families, lovers and friends; for the "worried well" (people who are seropositive on the HIV test or who have severe AIDS anxiety), for the bereaved, and for the community volunteers who do "frontline" work with persons with AIDS and AIDS related complex. Staff have co-led and supervised support groups, trained volunteers, and worked to develop a residence for people with AIDS. The center has not been funded for the staff costs or space used to implement this project. Negotiations are currently underway for the funding of program consultation services to expand the preventive emphasis at AIDS counseling and testing centers. In addition to developing a model to be implemented statewide, center staff will provide training and support for staff in these counseling and testing centers.

The *Survivors of Suicide Project* was initiated to meet the needs of family members and friends who are surviving the completed suicide of someone close to them. These survivors are at risk for pathological grief resolution and are vulnerable to biological, psychological, and interpersonal problems. Through monthly support group meetings facilitated by a professional and graduate trainees, survivors are offered education and support at no cost. Referrals for additional mental health services are made when appropriate. Much emphasis is placed on the use of the natural support system among group members between meetings.

Last year, member volunteers clocked over 300 hours of service providing written orientation materials to new group members, making direct phone contacts, and assisting with clerical tasks necessary to the maintainance of the group. Additionally, a regional conference is conducted yearly to permit persons from the larger region to benefit from didactic presentations and small group workshops. An average of 125 persons generally attend from New Jersey and neighboring states. Awards have been presented to media reporters who have shown exceptional sensitivity in their coverage of suicide stories.

As a result of major legislative appropriations for a variety of services, staff from the center's *Institute for Alzheimer's Disease and Related Disorders* have devoted thousands of hours to the provision of information, counseling, and support to reduce caregiver stress and prevent the breakdown of the family as the patient's major resource. Staff have provided technical assistance and educational services to caregiver support groups in the community and have developed a file on statewide specialized resource services for effective linkage of families to these much needed services.

Strengthening Caregivers

The center's *Suicide Prevention Project* has involved three, distinct services for school personnel: crisis intervention training, awareness training, and policy consultation. The crisis intervention training is conducted for special services staff through a 16-hour course which emphasizes identification, assessment, and referral. The awareness training improves recognition of warning signs of at-risk adolescents and helps school staff to identify internal and external resources for appropriate help. Last year, 2,010 school, health and human service professionals participated in the crisis intervention or awareness training. Increasingly, project staff have been called upon to provide consultation to school systems on the development of suicide prevention policies and procedures and to offer consultation (postvention) after there has been a completed suicide. The main emphasis of postvention services is to guide schools to adopt policies which will diminish contagion and to assist staff so they can be more responsive to students' needs. During the past year, 1,662 persons were provided these Postvention services. The center also participated in a demonstration project funded by the state where 512 school staff and parents were direct recipients of additional training, policy, and curriculum related consultation.

The Suicide Prevention Project is staffed by two full-time staff members with an additional four part-time staff members who provide services when needed. The project is currently supported through fees for service and state contracts. Staff members are seeking funding to conduct a more thorough evaluation of the crisis intervention training. To date, evaluation of all components of the project has been limited to consumer feedback and pre-post assessments of impact on knowledge, comfort, and perceived impact on skills. The results have been supportive of the model's efficacy.

Other preventive interventions have included mental health consultation to seventeen area nursery schools, day care centers, and Head Start programs in the catchment area. Thirty agencies in the county received program consultation and program evaluation assistance related to teenage pregnancy and parenting. In addition, organizational assessments were conducted with 33 agencies throughout four counties in central New Jersey that work with pregnant or parenting adolescents. Analysis of the assessment data determined what essential organizational factors were present in agencies which were more likely to conduct primary and secondary prevention services. Recommendations were made to state and local administrators regarding service delivery for pregnant and parenting teens. As another example, program consultation was offered to a community agency on the design, implementation, and evaluation of a child abuse and neglect program for the Hispanic community.

Ecological Interventions

Employee assistance services were provided to a number of New Jersey businesses and organizations. In addition to employee counseling and referral services, the center's employee assistance program offers ongoing management consultation to its employer-clients regarding human resource concerns, worksite health promotion, and the development of a positive organizational climate.

A staff member designed a radio broadcasted psychoeducational service for college campus radio stations. This preventive intervention presents taped dramatizations of problem situations typically encountered by college students (e.g., academic stress, interpersonal conflict, peer pressure to use alcohol or drugs). Using taped dramatizations, problem solving strategies and referral resources are presented. By providing this service on the campus radio, college administrators may help create a prosocial community environment where listeners learn the skills presented and apply these skills in their interpersonal relationships. An evaluation component is currently in development to determine whether the dramatizations and consultative message has a positive impact on listeners.

Social-Political Change

Many staff members are involved in consultative activities to create social policy and mental health service policy change. Staff have provided consultation to both the New Jersey Division on Alcoholism and the Division of Mental Health and Hospitals. Consultation has also been offered to several state departments regarding the program design of urban youth initiatives. In addition, the center's director and several staff have provided leadership on statewide task forces on suicide prevention and child abuse prevention.

Community Organization

A variety of advocacy activities have been undertaken related to the homeless, fair housing, neighborhood democracy, and racial justice. A Hispanic Community Health Council was organized to assess health needs and to provide health information on an ongoing basis to the Hispanic community. Finally, staff consulted with community advocacy groups such as the Concerned Citizens for Chronic Psychiatric Adults and the Shared Housing Association of New Jersey to establish new housing options, furnish apartments, and advocate around legislation impacting the mentally ill.

CONCLUSION

While there are many factors which have accounted for the successful development and management of prevention services at our center, the strength and continuity of leadership has been most important. The director of our center has been instrumental in creating and facilitating an organizational climate conducive to conducting prevention. The director's skills in strategic planning and advocacy efforts for prevention services in state and county service planning has also been essential. Strong leadership has also been important within the coordinating position for prevention services. Our prevention coordinators have exercised leadership that has been proactive rather than reactive to current and future funding and ideological trends. Sensitivity to organizational development issues has been helpful in assessing and intervening with potential internal obstacles to prevention program development.

While prevention coordinators need strong administrative skills, they also need a solid knowledge base in prevention theory, intervention, and applied research. Prevention staff members also need a strong theoretical background and knowledge base in conducting prevention and community-system work. Our director has recognized the need to hire coordinators and staff with an expertise in prevention services. For those individuals lacking in certain skill areas, they have been encouraged to seek out in-house or external personnel development and training to maintain and update their skills in the latest prevention technologies.

Finally, in order to have a successful prevention program, a center also needs to have a strong direct service component. Prevention services often act as a gatekeeper for clinical services. The provision of a variety of quality clinical services helps to facilitate a positive relationship between the prevention service specialists and the community they serve.

REFERENCES

Backer, T. E., & Levine, I. S. (1983). New directions in mental health consultation. *Consultation*, *3*, 12-20.

Bergner, L. L. (1981). The making of a consultation program. *Administration in Mental Health*, *8*, 237-247.

Bevilacqua, J. J. (1982). The changing federal-state human service system: Perspectives from a state commissioner of mental health and mental retardation. *Consultation*, *1*, 18-22.

Broskowski, A., & Baker, F. (1974). Professional, organizational, and social barriers to primary prevention. *American Journal of Orthopsychiatry*, *44*, 707-719.

Brown, V. B. (1983). Commentary. *Consultation*, *2*, 28-29.

Cherniss, C. (1977). Creating new consultation programs in community mental health centers: Analysis of a case study. *Community Mental Health Journal*, *13*, 133-141.

Davis, H. R. (1973). Change and innovation. In S. Feldman (Ed.), *The administration of mental health services*. Springfield, IL.: Charles C Thomas.

Davis, H. R., & Salasin, S. E. (1980). Change: Decisions and their implementation. In S. Feldman (Ed.), *The administration of mental health services* (2nd ed.). Springfield, IL: Charles C Thomas.

Erchul, W. P., & Backer, T. E. (1984). Recent developments in mental health consultation and education. *Consultation*, *4*, 57-59.

Ketterer, R. F., & Perkins, D. N. T. (August, 1977). *Factors affecting the development of consultation and education services in community mental health services*. Paper presented at the American Psychological Association Annual Convention, San Francisco.

Morgan, J. R. (in press). Applied community psychology: A ten-year field trial. In J. Rappaport & E. Seidman (Eds.), *Handbook of Community Psychology*.

Perlmutter, F., & Silverman, H. (1973). Conflict in consultation-education. *Community Mental Health Journal*, *9*, 166-122.

Price, R. H., & Politser, P. E. (1980). *Evaluation and action in the social environment*. New York: Academic Press.

Raber, M. F. (1984). Management of consultation and education programs in the community mental health center. *Administration in Mental Health*, *12*, 89-109.

Rossi, P. H. (1978). Issues in the evaluation of human service delivery. *Evaluation Quarterly*, *2*, 573-599.

Snow, D. L., & Newton, P. M. (1976). Task, social structure and social progress in the community mental health center movement. *American Psychologist*, *31*, 582-588.

Stanford, N. (1970). What ever happened to action research? *Journal of Social Issues*, *26*, 3-23.

Trickett, E. J., Kelly, J. G., & Vincent, T. A. (1985). The spirit of ecological inquiry in community research. In D. Susskind & D. Klien (Eds.), *Community research and action*. Cambridge. MA: Harvard University Press.

Twenty Years of Primary Prevention: Consultation, Education and Prevention at the Washtenaw County Community Mental Health Center

Ruth F. Schelkun

Washtenaw County Community Mental Health Center

SUMMARY. Throughout the two decades of the agency's existence, Consultation, Education and Prevention programming at the Washtenaw County Community Mental Health Center has developed, adapted, and survived during a number of major changes in agency mission, priorities, structures, and resources. Examples of services and products, a discussion of management issues, a look at the programs' relationship to theory, research, and practice, and a brief overview of the barriers and opportunities to such programming will provide an understanding of the many vicissitudes which C,E&P programs have faced since the original Federal staffing grants mandated these services as essentials among the offerings of comprehensive Community Mental Health centers.

Acknowledgment of valuable editorial assistance should be made to Robert Hess of the Riverwood Center in Benton Harbor, MI. Long term support and advice crucial to the growth and development of the Center's C,E&P programs have been provided by Saul Cooper, County Administrator and Director of the Washtenaw County Human Services Agency, by Lucy Ann Howard, Director of the Community Mental Health Division of the Washtenaw County Human Services Agency, and by Betty Tableman, Director of the Prevention Unit of the Michigan Department of Mental Health. Over the years, Michael Murphy has remained a valued colleague, active in planning and delivering the C,E&P services described here.

Requests for additional information should be addressed to the author at 3517 Terhune, Ann Arbor, MI 48104, or to Michael B. Murphy at the Washtenaw County Community Mental Health Center, 110 North Fourth Avenue, Ann Arbor, MI 48104.

The Washtenaw County Community Mental Health Center is a comprehensive community mental health center (CMHC), funded chiefly by the Michigan Department of Mental Health, through annual performance contracts which specify the services to be provided. As with most publicly supported CMHCs in the 1980s, most of these services are related to the process of deinstitutionalization, serving very helpless and disabled residents of the county. Within this context, the small Consultation, Education, and Prevention (C,E&P) Unit has managed to survive the changes brought about during the present decade and has maintained the C,E&P momentum which was developed in the 1970's under the agency's eight year federal staffing grant. A brief summary of the CMHC's history will disclose the context in which the C,E&P services have grown during the past twenty years of the organization's existence.

During the late 1960's, the community mental health movement developed a strong momentum, and CMHCs were established across the nation—hoping to attract generous funding through abundant, readily available federal staffing grants. One of five essential services for federally funded CMHCs was defined as "consultation and education (C&E)," the component most readily associated with prevention services. At about that time, several primary prevention pioneers joined the faculty of the University of Michigan in Ann Arbor, teaching the principles of C&E and of mental health prevention/promotion—in addition to serving on the steering committee or on the staff of the newly-established Washtenaw County Community Mental Health Center (WCCMHC). These community-oriented founders and early influencers of the WCCMHC included community psychologist and adjunct professor, Saul Cooper; James Kelly of the Department of Psychology; Tom Powell of the School of Social Work; William Morse and William Rhodes of the School of Education; Philip Margolis of Community Psychiatry; and Lucy Ann Howard of the School of Nursing. Later on, Richard Price became the Chair of the the newly-established Community Psychology department, continuing the relationship with the WCCMHC, and was joined by other members of University of Michigan departments interested in preventive aspects of mental health service delivery. During the height of the community mental health movement, graduate courses and seminars were taught in each of these departments, offering seminars in the theory and practice of consultation and mental health education—as well as in the more general issues associated with primary prevention programming. Over the years, the CMHC's university collaborations have continued and have spread to additional educational institutions.

Because of these beginnings, C&E activities were included among the earliest services developed and nurtured at the WC-CMHC—whose first director was Philip Margolis, a community psychiatrist. He was soon succeeded by the CMHC's long-term director, Saul Cooper, a well-known theoretician, promoter, and practitioner of C,E&P, and an APA Fellow in community psychology. When the agency was established in 1969, various C,E&P projects for community and caregiver systems were developed and fostered by the forementioned pioneers—for example, a district-wide school consultation project was spearheaded by James Kelly, a clergy consultation project was developed by Tom Powell, and a social services consultation project and a police consultation project were developed and supervised by William Rhodes. Later, these and other kinds of projects became ongoing elements of the WC-CMHC's "essential" consultation and education program, established and funded in the early 1970s under an eight year federal staffing grant. Because of its ongoing relationships with various university departments, both at the University of Michigan and nearby Eastern Michigan University, the C,E&P program was in close touch with the newly-developing concepts and practices in the field, and fostered graduate student internships, which enriched the C&E staffing resources while offering a cross-fertilization of theory and practice during the growth years of the 1970s.

Later, during the dry 1980s, when federal funding was no longer available to CMHCs for C,E&P programming, the capacity and momentum which had been established at WCCMHC enabled the continued development and adaptation of the Consultation, Education, and Prevention Unit—supported partly through a fee system but chiefly through funding which followed the priorities and guidelines of the Prevention Unit of the Michigan Department of Mental Health (Tableman, 1985). During the past two decades, the boundaries of the C,E&P program have been mostly influenced by changes in resources and the shifting priorities in the CMH domain, while the services have been varied and enriching, given the ongoing commitment to primary prevention goals, concepts, and practices by the agency's leadership, the Michigan Department of Mental Health, and successive boards of CMHC directors.

C,E&P SERVICES

Chiefly, the agency's C,E&P programs involve competency-building activities for caregivers, organizations, individuals at risk for various mental health related disabilities, the general public, and such general settings as neighborhoods and business districts. These activities are guided by the concepts, strategies, and principles of primary prevention in mental health, developed and promulgated by a number of pioneers in the field (Albee, 1982; Cooper & Hodges, 1983; Cowen, 1977,1985; Price et al, 1980). A brief summary of the categories of C,E&P services may highlight some of the ways that primary prevention goals are implemented at this CMHC:

Caregiver consultation. Following practices first developed by Gerald Caplan (1970), C,E&P staff offer both client-centered and consultee-centered consultation to such caregivers as teachers, police officers, day care personnel, parents, and others who may have difficulty understanding the thoughts, feelings, and behaviors of individuals for whom they are responsible. The goal of such consultation is to enhance the caregiver's skills in dealing with similar difficulties once the consultant is no longer present.

Program consultation. When a disabling pattern of behaviors is noted, C,E&P staff offer the next level of consultation highlighted by Caplan – assisting caregivers and their supervisors in designing and implementing positive environmental and programmatic changes. This level of consultation is designed to have further-reaching effects than caregiver consultation, and can be expected to continue its impact when consultees are replaced by others in their roles.

Administrative and organizational training and consultation. A rich literature in the field of organizational development has shown that dysfunctional organizational practices have negative effects on both personnel and clients of an agency, school, or business setting.

Therefore C,E&P staff offer consultation and training in such areas as participative problem solving, meetings management, organizational communication, organizational self-assessment, organizational restructuring, transitional management, supervisory skills, and time management. Although one-on-one administrative consultation has been emphasized by Caplan, various other strategies of consultation and training have been carefully conceptualized and put into practice by a large cohort of organizational development consultants (Lippitt & Lippitt, 1987; Schmuck & Runckel, 1985). Using organizational development practices over the years, C,E&P staff have maintained professional relationships with various agencies and organizations, adapting their services to individual need. These services have often been utilized as long-term interventions, which seek to strengthen, effectuate, and meliorate a variety of successive working and service delivery environments.

Networking, brokerage, and community resource development. Because C,E&P staff have extensive community contacts, they frequently serve as linkage agents for caregivers and informal community helpers. Their mobility within the county sensitizes them to become aware of new trends, unmet needs, and underserved populations. When this occurs, they may engage in a wide variety of approved community organization activities in order to assist in developing permanent new resources, many of which affect the quality of life for the community as a whole. Other such activities are directed toward assisting the support of deinstitutionalized populations served by the other CMHC programs. At times, in addition to consultating and training, the C,E&P staff may serve as temporary staffing for community-based programs during their early development; however, from the very start of their involvement CMHC staff are careful to plan the process for their orderly withdrawal.

In assisting with the development of new community resources, C,E&P staff have benefited from practices associated with the concept of empowerment. A number of community psychologists have offered important guidelines for this form of service delivery (Reiff & Riessman, 1965; Sarason, 1972; Rappaport, 1977; Kelly,1983; Gruber & Trickett, 1987). However, experience has highlighted a number of limitations on the empowering strategies suitable for the staff of a county bureaucracy. C,E&P priorities must be compatible with those of the county commissioners as well as of the CMHC's policy board; their services must not support confrontational or controversial activities; they must remove themselves from the political arena; and they must not allow personal values to lure them into taking sides when neighborhood or community conflict occurs. Although this list of caveats may seem daunting to activists who operate out of settings which permit more visible commitment and advocacy, our service history has shown that acceptable empowerment strategies and resource development activities can be implemented effectively, within our limitations.

Collaborative planning and programming. Wherever possible, C,E&P staff seek collaborative interventions—working with other human service agencies and community organizations—in both the planning and implementation phases of service delivery. Not only does this activity help to avoid waste and duplication, but it also averts the likelihood of developing turf wars and assists with the formation of alliances which enhance all of the CMHC's activities in the community.

Public and practitioner education. Educational activities of the C,E&P staff go well beyond the usual public information activities of the CMHC, with the aim of building participant skills which can be expected to result in a spectrum of primary prevention outcomes. Workshops in stress management, problem solving, and general habit change are examples of educational activities which conceptually can be expected to enrich participants' competencies and thereby enhance their coping abilities. Training-of-trainer consultations and workshops in these and other skills are offered in order to increase and improve the network of skilled educational and organizational development practitioners in the community at large.

Materials development and dissemination. When needed, C,E&P staff develop workshop handouts, informational booklets, and videotapes—making these available at low cost to other CMHCs, community agencies, and individual practitioners. These adjuncts to our consultation and training interventions enable us to develop consistency in programming, when a number of different practitioners with different styles and backgrounds deliver similar services. Some examples of offerings presently available or in development include (1) videotapes to train library staffs, business personnel, and human services in dealing with difficult and unusual behaviors or with eccentric individuals in the community, (2) a handbook for school administrators and pupil personnel staff to assist them in responding to traumatic events, (3) a pamphlet for parents and teachers to assist them in recognizing and adapting to maladaptive behaviors associated with intermittent hearing difficulties in children, and (4) a videotape for teachers, which assists them in implementing classroom methodologies for social problem solving which are included in the *Michigan Model for Comprehensive School Health* curriculum.

This variety of service activities demonstrates a rationale that encourages the C,E&P staff to become knowledgeable and to develop skills for a broad spectrum of primary prevention services, which can be expected to improve coping competencies and to enhance functioning, at all levels of the community.

A sample of some of the agency's C,E&P efforts in these areas during the past twenty years may indicate the scope of the agency's community-related prevention programming:

Community Resource Development: The Selected Neighborhoods Project (1971-1976)

This is an example of an extensive neighborhood empowerment and community resource development project which enabled the CMHC to take the lead in an early ecological intervention – sharing staff and other resources with a CMHC-facilitated community steering committee within a cluster of three contiguous low-income neighborhoods. Residents were seeking ways to prevent the spread of early neighborhood blight in 2,000 newly-built, low-income housing units. Using federal staffing grant resources and guided by a number of community organization and ecological principles which were just beginning to appear in the research literature, C,E&P staff facilitated the formation of a community resource advisory group and a Neighborhoods' Steering Committee – as well as a variety of functional task forces and committees. Project staff modeled a variety of roles and served as startup staff for such services as community program coordination, boys'/girls' club, a toddler drop-in center, HUD housing counseling, a pet control task force, a community newsletter, grant application, and a safety busing committee. Following this model, other agencies recruited residents for further programs and tasks, including a community health survey and the establishment of a community health clinic. Over time, many of these services, structures, and activities became permanently established. Finally, as planned, the selected neighborhoods obtained ongoing municipal resources, thereby retaining most of the community-based services, and WCCMHC prevention resources were phased out. The neighborhood resource model, established in those years, has since become the norm for municipally-funded services to these and similar neighborhoods in Ann Arbor.

More recently, the community resource development model of service delivery has facilitated such endeavors as (1) the development of Parish Partnerships—a countywide incorporated entity which supports preventive activities, using resources of various mental health agencies and the clergy and congregations of a number of religious organizations; (2) the development of Parents Together—an organization devoted to developing a range of prevention services for low-income, minority parents who live in a well-defined set of neighborhoods and whose members include local residents, housing project managers, and local minority clergy, as well as representatives of other agencies; and (3) the development of a Community Resource Center in a rural village whose service delivery system had been fragmented and uncoordinated, and whose need for coordination and resource development in prevention and other services was highlighted by the closing of one of the village's major industrial plants. Over the years, similar activities have permitted the WCCMHC to enable a neighborhood or other defined group to focus on and succeed in moving a vision of potential programming into actuality and permanence. We supply short-term resources and ongoing consultation—and phase back or out as the group builds its own identity and resource base.

Preventive Services to Schools

From the beginning, the CMHC has offered extensive, planned C,E&P programming to a number of the county's school districts.

The Willow Run School District Consultation Program (1970-1977), the Behavioral Science Education Project (BSEP) (1972-1979), and the present Quality of School Life (QSL) Program were developed and maintained as multi-level, systems-oriented, school-based prevention services. These programs reflect a major interest of the C,E&P program, offering a broad spectrum of consultative, collaborative, and educational services directed toward improving professional, organizational, and social problem-solving competencies, both in the classroom and within the caregiving organization.

Beginning with a core-group case consultation program for each elementary school in a low income community (Willow Run Project) and changing to a county-wide affective education focus (BSEP), programming has moved on to develop a multi-level (QSL) model for elementary schools, which is based on industry's quality circle/quality of work life participatory decision-making/team-building model. Using a classroom social competency curriculum (Schelkun, 1989), videotapes, and various handouts, staff members train administrators in participatory management concepts and methods, assist teachers to develop problem-solving quality circles in their elementary school classrooms; facilitate the development of staff involvement steering committees for schools; and assist with the development of family involvement units in parent-teacher organizations.

As a result of WCCMHC's long-term experience in this field, the Michigan Department of Mental Health recently commissioned the Washtenaw County C,E&P staff to create lessons for the now widely-used, state-sponsored *Michigan Model for Comprehensive Health Education* curriculum, and to train *Michigan Model* program coordinators, teachers, and the staff of other mental health centers in methods of developing children's social competency skills, which are highlighted in the curriculum.

Since 1972, as an adjunct to its school consultations, the C,E&P staff have created a School Crisis Response Team which delivers immediate consultation and educational interventions to school administrators and personnel during the often chaotic aftermath of death or serious accident which affects students, school personnel, or related families. Over the years, this service has created an interest and awareness in the county's school districts, so that it has been possible to develop a county-wide School Crisis Response Task

Force, with representation from many of the local districts, which is now developing policy and procedure manuals for responding to traumatic events within various school districts. Presently, as an outgrowth of this collaboration, the C,E&P staff are developing a general *School Crisis Response Manual* for school administrators and personnel.

Single-Need Response

Periodically, when a specific, compelling need arises in the county, the C,E&P unit collaborates with other WCCMHC units and with additional organizations, to respond to that need. The Community Support for the Homeless Project (1984-present) is an example of such a response. Like the more generalized community resource development projects, the CMHC's homeless project focuses on the development of new resources, consultation to affected settings, and community competency training strategies in order to serve a single, clearly established need—seeking and welcoming collaboration with other agencies and encouraging eventual independence from WCCMHC support wherever this is appropriate.

As an adjunct to efforts to encourage and develop competencies in nonprofessional volunteers and staffs of groups or agencies which serve the homeless, the C,E&P program has created training videotapes for managing difficult situations in public libraries, businesses, and community settings, as well as in programs which serve the homeless. Using these films, staff have worked toward community acceptance of the various street-persons' eccentricities by improving business' and caregivers' ability to deal with unusual, upsetting, or angry behaviors. In addition, C,E&P staff serve on community task forces for the development of affordable housing and for exploring other needs of this population and individuals at risk of homelessness.

Organizational Development (OD) (1972-present)

Since the early beginnings of the program, C,E&P staff have been encouraged to intervene at the systems level, whenever this is appropriate, assisting caregiving organizations to improve organizational practices where these affect the well-being of personnel or the delivery of services. Frequently, it has been possible to offer professional development training or case consultation as an initial intervention and later graduate to administrative consultation and training, with the goal of improving program and organizational effectiveness.

OD services have been delivered to a wide variety of organizations for—example, clergy and their congregations, police and legal-correctional agencies, day care centers, schools, service clubs, public service agencies, volunteer organizations, and other mental health agencies. The Quality of School Life program for school districts is an example of a major, system-wide organizational development intervention aimed at developing participative structures, concepts, and practices at all levels of a school district—including the elementary school classroom.

Collaborative Programming (1969-present)

From the beginning, the CMHC's C,E&P efforts have demonstrated values supporting shared ownership wherever this has been possible and appropriate—not an easy task, when preservation of strong boundaries has been the norm for most agencies' programs. For example, the C,E&P program offers stress management and habit change training modules, emphasizing cognitive/emotional skills, as part of Washtenaw County's WORKWELL program—a collaborative service whose lead agency is the Department of Public Health, which delivers health promotion services to personnel in local workplaces utilizing resources of various county agencies. We have actively participated in many collaborative projects sponsored by Parish Partnerships of Washtenaw County—an organization composed of representatives from various congregations and mental health agencies. We also collaborate in various ways with university-based prevention research projects, such as the federally funded Michigan Prevention Intervention Research (MPIRC) program (Price et al.,1985), and a state-funded Children of Divorce Project. In addition, C,E&P staff collaborate in undergraduate and graduate training in local universities—either as guest lecturers or as ongoing faculty for graduate level consultation courses, seminars, and practica. Recently, through funding from the Michigan Department of Mental Health, C,E&P staff have taken the initiative in the county to encourage the development and maintenance of new structures, which serve to coordinate the prevention activities of various county departments and human service agencies.

THE RESEARCH/PRACTICE LINK

C,E&P services work best when they combine the efforts of an interdisciplinary team. In order to maintain a broad set of skills and a variety of collegial relationships it is necessary, in this work, to have a broad-based, eclectic understanding of the research, theoretical, and practice literature of a variety of fields and professions. These include psychology, psychiatry, social work, education, organizational behavior and administration, nursing, school counseling, community development, family systems theory, and a variety of related areas. Following is a sample of the research and practice areas which have been essential to the C,E&P program:

- Prevention practice has required an up-to-date understanding of the *clinical/therapeutic literature*, since case consultation and brokering have frequently provided entry for eventual preventive programmatic and systemic interventions.
- The vast literature reflecting research, theories, and practical suggestions regarding types, methods, and strategies of *consultation* has provided an essential foundation for all our C,E&P activities. Approaches which relate to consultee-centered case, program, or administrative consultation, concepts involving community organization and ecological issues, and literature which focuses on organizational dynamics and social systems issues offer examples of research and theory which become increasingly important when activities are directed toward lasting change and stabilization in caregiver populations, community settings, and organizational systems.

In addition, specialized projects require a knowledge of more focused literature relating to specific issues. For example, the growing literature on the extent and effects of homelessness, industry's publications on quality of work life and other participatory decision-making approaches, education's widely disseminated literature on educational excellence and effectiveness, the broad-based literatures on social competency training, literature relating to the causes, assessment, and management of stress, and the literature associated with the adult learning model have all contributed to the success of our C,E&P programming over the years.

Unfortunately, the Washtenaw County C,E&P program has a sketchy history of implementing its own research and evaluation endeavors—since community mental health centers are rarely funded for any but the most rudimentary practices in this area. At times, graduate student interns have been able to match their needs with the evaluation needs of the program and have enabled us to collect and analyze data on a small scale. Recently, however, two years of Department of Mental Health funding for the Quality of School Life (QSL) program's classroom social competency intervention has included a fairly ambitious evaluation component, comparable to those otherwise funded efforts which have pioneered research in the area of children's social competency (Ojemann, 1969; Shure & Spivack, 1982; Gesten et al., 1982). Although data is still undergoing collection and analysis, this effort indicates that—when teachers educate and empower children in elementary school classrooms using a structured problem solving curriculum (Schelkun, 1989)—the group functions more effectively, classroom management becomes more participative, and the classroom climate becomes safer and more orderly. The class becomes more focused in its problem-solving activities, offers fewer ineffective or confusing strategies, and is far more likely to reach an appropriate solution to a typical interpersonal problem than untrained classrooms. In addition, problem solutions are more likely to involve appropriate proactive behaviors in the trained classrooms, while untrained groups are more likely to offer solutions involving inappropriate withdrawal or giving up. Data on individual outcomes are still being analyzed; however, teacher reports and consultant diaries indicate that individual competencies follow a similar pattern.

C,E&P program evaluations for most interventions usually involve client satisfaction questionnaires or interviews (usually for educational presentations), consultant logs, and the informal, but politically effective good will, word-of-mouth affirmations, and thank you letters which are so important to the survival of applied programs which originate from a service base. Under the present funding and accountability circumstances, for good or ill, program evaluation is far more likely to involve anecdotal and testimonial responses than the more objective formal procedures which have been discussed in the literature (Mannino & MacLennan, 1978; Price et al., 1980).

MANAGEMENT ISSUES

Managing a small, low-budget prevention program which is embedded in a mental health center whose primary mission is treatment, support, and habilitation has presented numerous difficulties from the beginning. A wide range of issues and suggested solutions or guidelines to solve the numerous management problems have been discussed at length elsewhere (Broskowski et al., 1978; McPheeters, 1981; Schelkun et al., 1979; Schelkun et al., 1981). This paper will indicate ways that a few salient management issues have been dealt with in Washtenaw County.

PLACE IN THE ORGANIZATION

It is difficult to face the fact that there is no comfortable place in the organization for a program as marginal as C,E&P has been since its inception. No matter how much the program is valued by its leadership and by the community, it remains so poorly funded, compared to other units within the agency, that it is always seen as being out of balance with the other units in the agency when it attempts to achieve the necessary recognition, resources, power, communication opportunities, decision-making linkages, and other assets which are necessary for it to function and survive. Directors of the agency never quite know where to put it, when redesigning the chart of organizational structure. Moreover, there has always been the associated problem of intra-agency boundary-spanning. Staff members of other units necessarily perform some C,E&P functions, in addition to their major responsibilities, and their unit managers are rarely willing or able to relinquish the direction of their activities to the C,E&P manager or supervisor.

At Washtenaw CMHC, the C,E&P program has moved about in the agency during the past twenty years. When services were delivered in duplicate units within three separate geographical areas, each unit had its own C,E&P subprogram – sometimes with its own supervisor and sometimes supervised by the program's general manager. When this structure became too fragmented, a central C&E director coordinated the C&E functions of the three units in a modified matrix management design. Later, when the agency changed its structure to countywide functional units, most of the identified C,E&P functions were placed in the present separate Community Services unit – with various treatment and rehabilitation units delivering some additional C,E&P services when this seemed more practical.

Closely related to the problem of where to place the programming has been the dilemma of administrative oversight – to whom should the C,E&P activities report? At Washtenaw, at different times, the same C&E manager/supervisor has reported successively to two program managers at once, to a single manager, to the Director of the agency, to the Associate Director, and finally, to the Director's office – with direct access to both the Director and Associate Director. This arrangement has given the C,E&P unit equal management status with the larger program units – with similar control over program budget, participation in administrative decisions, and much more predictable "dotted line" relationships with other program managers.

FUNDING

In the 1980s, CMHCs have had to diversify their methods of funding their various endeavors; for prevention programming, that includes searching out methods of increasing the base by collecting fees for a variety of services. This has meant considering ability to pay as well as need when developing programs and setting priorities for the use of resources. Using a "sliding scale" rationale similar to that for treatment programs, Washtenaw's C,E&P offerings to more affluent private sector recipients have helped support some additional services to those with limited ability to pay. Locally, there is heavy competition to develop and deliver services which show a strong ability to generate funds (for example, employee assistance programs and stress management workshops), so there is continual pressure to stay ahead of the game in program selection, marketing, staffing credibility, quality of programming, and networking.

The search for local, consumer-generated dollars has secondary benefits: it forces the program staff out of their comfort zone—requiring them to maintain close ties to various levels in the community, to remain current, and to build mutually beneficial coalitions in order to reduce the negative effects of excessive competition. Among these negative effects are the need to spend resources in marketing endeavors when these might otherwise be used for service delivery; the discouragement of *pro bono* activities, in favor of those which can bring in adequate fees, the lack of research and program evaluation since these are rarely supported by fees, the departure of skilled staff for more prestigious or more lucrative work, and the disappearance from the field of practitioners who lack competitive energy and motivation, but who have other useful abilities.

In addition, since C,E&P capacity is built on a base of public funding, there are a number of restrictions on the ability to use fees to develop further programming; consequently, the growth of separately-funded activities is slow and the total amounts raised each year are small. Practically speaking, what this means is that while the search for "outside dollars" continues, some promising programs have been abandoned because the marketplace could not support them, some activities have been working toward self-support, and the majority of programs still require the continued support of the Department of Mental Health's Prevention dollars.

STAFFING

Presently, the C,E&P unit's staffing is managed both with permanent and contractual staffing. This split-staffing design permits a functional balance between the competing needs of stability and flexibility in programming. The unit director and two additional full-time staff members are responsible for planning, supervising, and delivering the basic prevention functions of the Community Services Unit, while a host of other services are purchased from a variety of different vendors as specific skills and services are needed.

Washtenaw County is uniquely provided with credible, skilled entrepreneurs whose talents fit the array of prevention interventions provided by the program. Staff members are encouraged to network actively within the various professional organizations which relate to the field (for example, their own specific professional affiliations, the American Society for Training and Development and the Michigan Organization Development Network); therefore, it has been relatively easy to locate short-term staffing resources when these are needed.

MANAGEMENT INFORMATION

In a small unit, which represents less than one per cent of the agency's budget, there is little funder support for the detailed information and planning system which has been recommended in the literature (Broskowski et al., 1978). For a few years, while a federal staffing grant was in effect, the Prevention Unit of the Michigan Department of Mental Health funded the CMHC to develop and demonstrate a sophisticated management information system for all C,E&P activities provided by any personnel. Using this system, for several years, it was possible for us to examine a monthly printout indicating who did what, for whom, for how long, and when—noting every recipient agency or group, the amount of staff time dedicated to each activity, which unit delivered the service, the types of service delivered, the number of recipients, and other facts helpful for planning and monitoring programs. Comprehensive files were developed for recipient organizations, and these were kept up to date—much as treatment files are kept and supervised. Since that time, however, the agency's management information system has been adapted to the reporting requirements set forth by the Department of Mental Health and other sources of funding and reimbursement. Because the treatment and habilitation programs represent the bulk of the agency's funding, the C,E&P reporting system has been streamlined to offer only the small amount of aggregated information necessary for reports to be written and to assure fiscal accountability.

PROCESS ISSUES

Despite the frequent changes that have occurred during the relatively short life span of the Washtenaw CMHC, C,E&P service capacity has developed in a remarkably linear fashion when we view the vicissitudes of similar program building in many other CMHCs. There have been no major discontinuities in the range, kinds, and flexibility of services—even at a time when most staff members were reassigned and the quantity of such services was severely reduced during the CMHC's shift in service toward issues of deinstitutionalization and during Michigan's fiscal recession in 1979 and 1980. Consequently, the program has been able to maintain the capacity to attract new resources, when these have become available, and to maintain consumer trust in the predictability, quality, and consistency of its service offerings.

When others ask, "How did you do it?," the list of likely factors that led to C,E&P success is far too long to discuss in detail here. However, it may be helpful to consider a few noteworthy issues.

CONTINUITY OF ADMINISTRATIVE SUPPORT AND STAFF SOPHISTICATION

First of all, we've been lucky! The agency has had only three directors during its lifespan: Philip Margolis, Saul Cooper, and more recently Lucy Ann Howard—all of whom are nationally known as contributors to and supporters of the values of the community mental health movement in general—and of consultation, education, and prevention services in particular. Thus, the C,E&P programs have maintained a consistent mission, theoretical base, and source of administrative support, throughout several agency reorganizations. In addition, a core of C,E&P staff—well grounded in both theory and practice—has stayed with the agency, providing a constant nucleus for C,E&P training and activity, even when staff has been assigned to other units. We have also been fortunate in the stability of leadership at the state level; Betty Tableman has been the Director of the Prevention Services Unit of the Michigan Department of Mental Health since the unit's inception; consequently, there have been no discontinuities in our relationship to the department. This fact was crucial to the development and survival of C,E&P programming in Michigan, once the federal dollars were no longer available. Washtenaw CMHC has been actively represented on the Department of Mental Health's Prevention Advisory Council, which meets regularly with Ms. Tableman to develop and maintain common goals, values, practices, and service strategies in CMHCs across the state, as well as to communicate with and advise the department in areas of program development and policy formation (Smith & Hess, 1985).

We have also been responsive to the major mission of the CMHC. Although the major thrust of C,E&P programming continues to focus on primary prevention activities, we have developed effective methods for improving community acceptance of the CMHC's deinstitutionalization efforts. Consultation and staff/community education in dealing with difficult situations have been delivered to numerous public and private settings impacted by the presence of homeless individuals or those whose eccentric behavior is perceived as frightening or confusing. These services have been enthusiastically received and have enabled CMHC administrators and board members to perceive the C,E&P unit as a relevant adjunct to other program units of the CMHC.

BROAD COMMUNITY INVOLVEMENT AND WIDE SCOPE OF SERVICE

It has been the practice of C,E&P staff to "Never say 'No,'" when approached with a request—either from within the CMHC or from the community. If we can't provide a requested service, we assist in the search for other providers or in designing an alternate approach which may better meet the need. The program has never been static, since the community's needs keep changing. The major successes of the program have arisen from its broad range of community contacts and the wide scope of staff skills and legitimized service activities which have enabled C,E&P staff to react quickly and appropriately to requests and to foresee and meet needs for future services, sometimes even before services are requested.

COLLABORATIVE RELATIONSHIPS AND COMMUNITY RESOURCE BUILDING

From the beginning, empire building has been discouraged and collaborations have been fostered – by the Michigan DMH Prevention Unit, as well as by the leadership of the CMHC. This approach has required considerable effort in coordinating efforts with others who have often been reinforced for more proprietary behaviors; however, the result has enabled us to function more effectively and to avoid confusing the recipients of service, by avoiding the kind of battlefield milieu which often exists when various uncoordinated agencies attempt to deliver similar services to the same groups of recipients. This enabling approach has also kept us from getting bogged down in delivering the same services to the same site over a long period of time; we are freed up to service the leading edge of need, because specific C,E&P services have been shared or given away. After a setting has received a concentrated amount of service for a period of time, our activities become less frequent and ongoing relationships become more collegial and collaborative. Our staff can then be re-assigned to other sites or new activities without losing the ongoing services which are now appropriately supported in other ways.

CROSS TRAINING AND SYSTEMATIZING WHAT WORKS

All members of the C,E&P unit are trained to understand and carry out a full range of activities in a variety of settings. Each staff member is given responsibility for a specific set of activities and for assuring that at least one other member of the unit is able to provide backup whenever this is necessary. We are able to do this because we have a small team of flexible individuals whose norms support cross training, interactive problem solving, and a sense of team ownership for all activities and outcomes. In addition, we develop systematic approaches to service development and delivery – creating handouts, handbooks, training videotapes, detailed workshop outlines, and the like whenever we find a method that works. This enables us to contract a number of services to providers who are not regular members of the C,E&P staff, without sacrificing control over content and methodology.

ATTITUDES, BEHAVIORS, AND PERSONAL CHARACTERISTICS

Washtenaw's C,E&P staff display a set of behaviors, characteristics, and attitudes which are helpful for all professionals but which are crucial for those who are out in the community most of the time, who have little on-site opportunity to mingle with their CMHC colleagues, whose budget is small, and whose services are often seen as marginal to the "real" functions of the CMHC. Their marginality is an asset to the organization since they are useful as boundary spanners, both within the CMHC and in the community. They must maintain a reputation for good judgement, confidentiality, discretion, flexibility, objectivity, and general helpfulness within their own organization, as well as with client systems in the community.

In practice, this means that they do not take sides in the many political and controversial situations that arise in the various subcultures within the CMHC as well as in community settings. Since any setting in the county is a potential client system of the C,E&P unit, C,E&P staff cannot join colleagues or friends who might criticize their own or other agency's practices, engage in political advocacy, or take a public stand on a controversial issue.

In addition to knowing how to educate and consult with others in specific content areas, the C&E practitioner needs an exceptional amount of resilience, self esteem, discretion, modesty, respect for cooperative endeavors, ability to learn new concepts and to continue to grow professionally, interpersonal skill, and a consistent problem-solving approach to all difficult situations. Our C,E&P staff develops and maintains these characteristics beyond the initial staff selection process by developing and nurturing team norms which support these attitudes and behaviors.

KEEPING UP WITH THE FIELD

The field of service delivery in consultation, education, and prevention is quite volatile. Because consultants and community educators are constantly interacting with many layers of the community and with other service providing agencies, they are often the first to note the emergence of new needs or opportunities for service. In order to remain responsive to such needs, practitioners must stay in touch with others in the field or in relevant research programs, who may have developed information or innovative approaches which address the challenges they encounter. Members of our C,E&P staff are encouraged to maintain active membership in a variety of professional organizations, to attend and present at conferences, to publish and disseminate information and materials from our successful programs, and to maintain a small library of relevant reprints and other publications.

DISAPPOINTMENTS AND DIFFICULTIES

It has always been difficult to find ways to cope with the fact that C,E&P practitioners never really belong in any of their workaday settings. They are guests in the places where they consult with and educate others; they are rarely on location at the CMHC, where they must protect their reputations, turf, and resources in an organization where their colleagues are more often to be found at the office; they perceive that their service unit never fits comfortably within the structure of the CMHC; and they must continually prepare to leave those outside settings where they are accepted and respected moving on to others where they must once again prove themselves. Many of our difficulties and disappointments, over the years, have been related to our marginality in the organization and in the community.

Some disappointments and difficulties have arisen because of the changing economy and the many changes in the funding sources and legitimation of C,E&P activities. From time to time, we have lost programs, staff, funding, and other supports for valued activities. One of the most difficult losses has been the serious depletion of our network of colleagues following the abrupt end to federal support for C&E activities in the many CMHCs across the state and nation. Although we have been among the fortunate CMHCs to have maintained a viable C,E&P unit, many others have not been able to do so, and this has led to a serious diminution of activity and cross-fertilization in the field. Our local universities now offer far less training for professionals in C,E&P activities, fewer professional publications offer research findings associated with successful consultation and community education practices, and we have few opportunities to hobnob with knowledgeable colleagues. Even when such opportunities are available, limited funding and small staffing makes it difficult to take time out to keep up with other C,E&P practitioners.

In addition, the present shortage of research and credible evaluation in the field have made it difficult to validate the considerable gains which practitioners see occurring in their work. Very few of us are encouraged to engage in the kinds of action research that would be likely to support widespread application of successful programs. Consequently, we are caught in a constant "Catch-22" situation: because funds for research and program evaluation are rarely adequate when we demonstrate new approaches, we continue to be told that C,E&P activities haven't proved themselves and therefore are not supportable on any large scale.

CONCLUSION

In sum, the C,E&P program of the Washtenaw County Community Mental Health Center has survived the many organizational and economic vicissitudes of the past twenty years to remain a viable service component throughout the full period of the agency's existence. In the volatile C,E&P marketplace, this has meant that our staff and most of our contractual colleagues have had to become knowledgeable and adaptable professional generalists, capable of adding, changing, and deleting effective service products fairly rapidly. Recognition comes slowly, however. Just recently, for twenty years of service, Washtenaw's Consultation, Education, and Prevention Unit became the first recipient of the Henry V. McNeill Award – given annually by the Community Psychology Division of the American Psychological Association to honor innovative community-based prevention efforts in the mental health field. Despite the many difficulties and challenges, there are many intrinsic rewards in our varied and busy days, and even though there are more traditional, remunerative, and more predictable ways to earn a living, Washtenaw's C,E&P practitioners consider themselves fortunate to be doing what they do in their work.

REFERENCES

Albee, G. (1982). Preventing psychopathology and promoting human potential. *American Psychologist*, *37*, 1043-1050.

Broskowski, A., Driscoll,J., & Schulberg, H.C. (1978). A management information and planning system for indirect services. In C. Attkisson, W.A. Hargreaves, & M.J. Horowitz (Eds.), *Evaluation of human service programs*. New York: Academic Press.

Caplan, G. (1970). *The theory and practice of mental health consultation*. New York: Basic Books.

Cooper, S. (1974). Role differentiation as a dimension in community diagnosis. *American Journal of Community Psychology*, *2*, 113-117.

Cooper, S. & Hodges, W. (1983). *The mental health consultation field*. New York: Human Sciences Press.

Cowen, E.L. (1985). Person-centered approaches to primary prevention in mental health: Situation-focused and competence enhancement. *American Journal of Community Psychology*, *13*, 31-48.

Cowen, E.L. (1977). Baby-steps toward primary prevention. *American Journal of Community Psychology*, *5*, 1-22.

Gesten, E.L., Rains, M.H., Rapkin, B.D., Weissberg, R.P., Flores de Apocada, R., Cowen, E.L., & Bowen, R. (1982). Training children in social problem-solving competencies: A first and second look. *American Journal of Community Psychology*, *10*, 95-115.

Gruber, J., & Trickett, E. J. (1987). Can we empower others? The paradox of empowerment in the governing of an alternative public school. *American Journal of Community Psychology*, *15*, 353-371.

Kelly, J. G. (1983). Consultation as a process of creating power: an ecological view. In S. Cooper & W. Hodges (Eds.), *The mental health consultation field*. New York: Behavioral Sciences Press.

Lippitt, N., & Lippitt, R. (1987). *The consulting process in action* (Rev. ed.). LaJolla, CA: University Associates.

Mannino, F.V., & MacLennan, B.W. (1979). *Monitoring and evaluating mental health consultation and education services*. Washington: Department of Health, Education, and Welfare.

McPheeters, H.L. (Ed.). (1981). *Definitions for prevention/promotion services in mental health*. Atlanta, GA: Southern Regional Education Board.

Ojemann, R. H. (1969). Incorporating psychological concepts in the school curiculum. In H. P. Clarizio (Ed.), *Mental health and the educative process*. Chicago: Rand-McNally.

Price, R., House, J., & Gordus, J. (1985). Exploring work as an arena for prevention research: The Michigan Prevention Research Center *Prevention in Human Services, 3/4*, 3-11.

Price, R.H., Ketterer, R.F., Bader, B.C., & Monahan, J. (Eds.). (1980). *Prevention in community mental health: Research, policy, and practice*. Beverly Hills, CA: Sage Publications.

Rappaport, J. (1977). *Community psychology: Values, research and action*. New York: Holt, Rinehart & Winston.

Reiff, R., & Riessman, F. (1965). The indigenous nonprofessional: A strategy of change in community action and community mental health programs. *Community Mental Health Journal*, Monograph No.1.

Sarason, S. (1972). *The creation of settings and the future societies*. San Francisco: Jossey-Bass.

Schelkun, R. (1989). *The classroom cooperation curriculum: Improving school and classroom climate through pupil involvement in problem solving with people*. Ann Arbor, MI: Human Networks.

Schelkun, R., Snow, D., Swift, C., & Cooper, S. (1981). *Recommended policies and procedures for consultation and education (C&E) services within community mental health systems/agencies*. Washington: National Council of Community Mental Health Centers.

Schelkun, R., Ravlin, M., & Haight, P. (1979). *Systematizing CMH-based consultation: Looking to the 1980's*. Paper presented at the 87th Annual Meeting of the American Psychological Association, New York City.

Schmuck R.A., & Runckel, P.J. (1985). *The handbook of organization development in schools* (3rd ed.). Palo Alto, CA: Mayfield.

Shure, M., & Spivack, G. (1982). Interpersonal problem-solving in young children: A cognitive approach to prevention. *American Journal of Community Psychology, 10*, 341-356.

Smith, F., & Hess, R. (1985). The role of the prevention advisory committee in Michigan. *Prevention in Human Services, 3*, 13-19.

Tableman, B. (1985). Overview of Michigan prevention programming. *Prevention in Human Services, 3*, 3-11.

Developing Prevention Programming in a Large Nonprofit Service Agency

Thomas A. Duke

St. Paul Area Council of Churches

Eugene S. Urbain

Amherst H. Wilder Foundation

SUMMARY. The Amherst H. Wilder Foundation has established prevention as one of its areas of emphasis and has created an interdisciplinary planning team to develop programming initiatives and to provide resources to other programs and organizations interested in prevention. A rationale for selecting new program initiatives has been developed as well as a funders guide. New initiatives include an interagency project to provide social support to parents under stress, a family wellness project, and consultation to neighborhood-based citizen action groups concerned about social problems. Attention is also being given to collaborative community planning and policy development in support of preventive approaches.

The Amherst H. Wilder Foundation is a large, endowed social service organization serving the four-county St. Paul metropolitan area with direct mental health services for children and families,

---

Thomas A. Duke is the former director of Community Care Resources and Prevention Programs at The Amherst H. Wilder Foundation, 919 Lafond Avenue, St. Paul, MN 55104. He is currently the Executive Director of the St. Paul Area Council of Churches. Eugene S. Urbain, is a staff psychologist with The Wilder Foundation. He works part-time in the Child Guidance Center and is Director of the Parent Outreach Project of the Wilder Foundation's Prevention Planning Team.

Reprints may be obtained from Eugene S. Urbain, Amherst H. Wilder Foundation, 919 Lafond Avenue, St. Paul, MN 55104.

comprehensive services for the elderly, and housing management services. The foundation also provides services to other nonprofit organizations in order to help them be more effective in providing services to needy populations. These services to organizations include management support, a conference and retreat center, and consultation and training regarding social support and prevention programming. A large research department serves both Wilder programs and outside nonprofit agencies. The Wilder Foundation has a long history of responding to the needs of disadvantaged people in its service area. Many innovative program efforts have been initiated in its nearly 80 years of operation. While many of these have been primarily remedial in nature, addressing illness or symptoms of a breakdown in individual or family functioning with treatment resources, some have also been preventive in that they have served to strengthen the resourcefulness of various populations—both to promote their health and welfare and to prevent the onset or duration of various disorders or problems.

Within the area of child and family mental health, several programs fit a traditional concept of preventive or early intervention efforts: a public playground/recreation program; a motivational tutorial program (college students volunteering to tutor school aged children); a youth-work program; and the Child Guidance Center (and its four branch offices), which since its origin has aimed to provide early intervention in order to prevent adult psychosocial disorder. The specific, long-term preventive impact of such programs has not been researched, and funding priorities have permitted only the Child Guidance Center to continue in operation.

Another program at the Wilder Foundation which has claimed prevention as a major operating theme and which continues in operation is the Community Care Resources (CCR) Program. The preventive thrust of this program is evident in the following examples of CCR projects:

- Support group development (e.g., "We Care" mutual-help for separated/divorced, grief groups for widowed persons and parents of deceased children, Parents Anonymous, parent support groups, caregiver groups).

- Development of neighborhood support systems in a mobile home park to aid parents and prevent child abuse.
- "Befriender" training, i.e., training lay persons to function as caregivers in their community or religious congregation by offering social support to persons experiencing various family or personal crises and stress.
- Providing staff for the Minnesota Chapter of the National Committee for the Prevention of Child Abuse in order to help conduct various prevention activities, such as messages in mass media and information for new parents ("Pierre the Pelican" child development newsletters).
- Providing a resource center (clearinghouse) for information, training, and consultation about self-help groups (Minnesota Mutual Help Resource Center).
- Training refugee natural helpers (community leaders, clergy, extended family members, healers, social service workers) to enhance their effectiveness as a vital part of Southeast Asian refugees' support systems.

RATIONALE FOR PREVENTION PROGRAMMING AT WILDER

Only in the last few years, however, has a prevention planning and program development effort been explicitly and intentionally organized and staffed. The theme of prevention had surfaced occasionally in planning and policy discussions at Wilder since a 1975 board-staff conference. At this conference, prevention was listed as an area of indirect service to which increased commitment should be made. The theme of prevention was again emphasized at Wilder's 1983 Board-Staff Conference as a part of a discussion of children's needs and programming. Information from a Young Adult Needs Assessment Survey conducted by the Wilder Research Center pointed to the vulnerability of young single mothers in terms of a lack of basic material needs, low levels of educational attainment, and an inability to find employment and achieve financial independence. Information on children from these single parent families (an increasing proportion of all children) suggested that they might be less well-equipped for a successful transition to adulthood. As a

Wilder Research Center report pointed out: "The number and proportion of children living in poverty is increasing . . . The community has a vested interest in the welfare of children from single parent families and should strive to insure that their needs are not neglected. Attending to the needs of these children implies support for single parents in their role as parents (Amherst H. Wilder Foundation, 1984)."

Another topic in the 1983 board-staff conference was a concern to find effective ways to address the problems related to increasing levels of reported child maltreatment, preferably using a preventive approach. Later that year, the staff of Community Care Resources submitted a proposal to the Wilder administration and Board of Directors requesting funding to initiate a long-term, major prevention planning effort. Further elements of rationale cited in the proposal included: (1) the lack of adequate professional treatment resources to serve the needs indicated by the high rates of abuse, neglect, chemical dependence, marital disruption, and children being raised in poverty; (2) the lack of significant attention or commitment to prevention programming by county, state, and federal policymakers; (3) interest on the part of Wilder staff; (4) funding available from The National Institute for Mental Health (NIMH) for prevention intervention research centers; and (5) the unique capacity of an organization like Wilder to combine research staff, clinical programs, credibility in the community, capacity to influence other service providers and policymakers, and a capable, motivated staff operating in a "services to organizations" mode.

Criteria and strategies for selecting specific prevention approaches were included in the original proposal in order to help the Wilder Board understand how the Prevention Planning Project would proceed. Criteria for decision-making were proposed as follows:

1. Knowledge of existing data base from research on various preventive interventions.
2. Cost-effectiveness considerations.
3. Level of willingness of relevant systems to cooperate or invest in preventive-oriented changes.
4. Resource availability (particularly regarding sustainability of an intervention program after the initial demonstration phase).

5. Capacity to measure results of particular interventions.
6. Capacity to assess risk within large populations and to gain access to at-risk sub-populations.
7. Capacity to be culturally sensitive in working with ethnic groups and disadvantaged groups.
8. Appeal to supporting audiences/groups.
9. Value judgments of funders/policy-makers about target populations and problems to be addressed.

The following strategies were suggested as a guide for planning specific interventions:

1. Pick a problem focus of interest to key actors and decision-makers.
2. Link closely with treatment providers for insights, guidance, support, and credibility.
3. Move, step by step, from current investment in treatment services to target groups which are "most at risk," to those "somewhat at risk," and eventually to the promotion of wellness for major general populations.
4. Build on previous and currently existing preventive interests in the community, in clinical settings, and in other agencies with a focus on prevention-oriented activities, (e.g., public health nursing and early childhood and family education in the schools).
5. Look for ways to develop untapped resources to finance, operate, and support prevention efforts (e.g., volunteer efforts, making low-cost changes in services of established agencies, pooling of resources, etc.).

The Prevention Planning Project proposal was funded by the Wilder Board in 1984 for an initial year with additional funding to be reviewed annually, based in part on success in attracting additional outside funding.

DESCRIPTION

Following the approval of the proposal for the Prevention Planning Project the Director of the Community Care Resources program was authorized to spend approximately one-third time to organize a Prevention Planning Team and initiate the project's activities. The following sections describe various aspects or subprojects which have been part of or have grown out of the Prevention Planning Project during its four years of existence.

Prevention Planning Team

At the outset of the project, an interdisciplinary team of Wilder staff was established to help guide and implement the project. The Prevention Planning Team was composed of the project director (pastoral counselor), a member of the Wilder Research Center staff (sociologist), a clinician from the Child Guidance Center (psychologist), and two trainers from Community Care Resources (a community psychologist and an educator).

The team met twice monthly to coordinate planning, discuss conceptual frameworks for prevention development, plan for library resource acquisition, and develop recommendations for specific programs/activities. Team members attended relevant conferences/meetings, contacted experts nationally, read different areas of literature, and shared as much information as possible with other team members.

Parent Outreach Project

The first major demonstration program growing out of the Prevention Planning Project is the Parent Outreach Project (POP), operated out of Wilder's Division of Services to Children and Families. POP is an interagency collaborative effort to link volunteer "parent befrienders" and professional service providers with parents who are pregnant or have infants under 12 months, where various factors suggest the family is under stress and at risk for parent-child problems. The project's major goal is preventing breakdown of parent-child relationships and child maltreatment by building on family strengths early in the life cycle.

Collaborating in the project are the Ramsey County Public Health Nursing Service, Ramsey Community County Human Services (Volunteer Services Department), and the Early Childhood Family Education programs of three local school districts in Ramsey County. Wilder staff provide planning, organizing, and research coordination, and share in the training and coordination of the volunteer befrienders. Public health nurses, acting as case managers, work closely with the county human services volunteer coordinator to match befrienders with appropriate families. Befrienders serve as: (a) friendly listeners, providing friendship and emotional support to the parents; (b) linking agents to help parents strengthen their own support networks and access community resources such as Early Childhood Family Education programs; and (c) informal role models for dealing with day-to-day issues of parenting and parent-child interaction.

The key ideas behind the demonstration project are (a) to build on family strengths early in the life cycle, (b) to use a collaborative approach with professionals and volunteers working in a team approach, (c) to provide services through a series of neighborhood-based implementation teams, (d) to coordinate services across agencies/disciplines for the benefit of the families involved, and (e) to contribute research data of national significance. The project is expanding on a neighborhood-by-neighborhood basis, respecting the uniqueness of individual neighborhoods and making sure that necessary groundwork and networking are done to gain proper entry and obtain the cooperation and sponsorship of important local groups in a particular neighborhood.

Following an initial one-year small scale pilot stage, federal funding for a three-year demonstration effort was granted for the project from the Division of Maternal and Child Health, U.S. Public Health Service, as a Special Project of Regional and National Significance. Each collaborating agency also makes a thirty percent in-kind contribution of services to the demonstration project as an "investment" in prevention. The full project demonstration effort (approximately three years) will be conducted with approximately 60 families. A second group of 60 families will serve as a comparison group, receiving standard nursing care. Evaluation will consist of the two groups of the parents being compared on measures of parent-child interaction, home environment, social network support, child protection reports, and child development. A cost-benefit analysis will be conducted following final data collection.

Funders' Guide

As the Wilder Foundation and the Prevention Planning Team considered beneficial ways to invest in prevention programming, a decision was made to attempt to turn the process of analysis and decision-making into a resource for other organizations facing similar choices. The result was a formulation by the Prevention Planning Team of a project entitled "A Funder's Guide to Prevention Planning in the Human Services." The project's purpose was to assist funders—both private and public—and policymakers by providing an analysis and critical overview of a number of prevention approaches in the human services. The specific objectives of the Funder's Guide project were as follows:

1. To provide clarification of the prevention concept as it applies to human services.
2. To provide a "state of the art" overview of prevention programming in selected problem areas of current interest (adolescent chemical abuse, poor school performance or failure; child maltreatment, and adolescent pregnancy).
3. To develop a set of working guidelines for use in evaluating proposals for prevention programs.

The objectives of the project were to be accomplished by reviewing relevant research literature, working with an advisory group and occasional roundtable focus groups composed of funders from different organizations, and convening a conference (April 1988) to discuss the project's findings with recognized professionals and funders from throughout Minnesota. The conference was held as planned, and products of the project include the Funders' Guide Manual containing definitions and guidelines for reviewing prevention program proposals for use by human service funders, board members, planners, and administrators; also, a full report of project findings is available in the form of a series of extended topical review papers.[1]

The project was implemented by staff of Wilder's Prevention Planning Team, with representation from both the Wilder Research Center and the Community Care Resources program, with the assistant director of the research center taking the lead role.

Other Wilder Prevention Initiatives

The Prevention Planning Team came early to the conclusion that collaborative, inter-organizational and grassroots efforts are very significant in many effective prevention efforts. Staff of Wilder's Community Care Resources had had previous experience in at least two projects dealing with the support and development of natural helping networks at a neighborhood level. One project aimed at reduction of child abuse in a mobile home park by identifying and supporting natural helpers and leaders; another aimed at identifying and reaching out to isolated elderly persons in urban neighborhoods by recruiting and supporting volunteer block workers to deliver a newsletter which addressed the needs of elderly persons and gave the volunteer an opportunity to develop relationships with elderly persons. In order to build on this experience, the Prevention Planning Team convened a "neighborhood development interest group" open to Wilder staff and a number of community persons. The group met bimonthly for 2 years to discuss various aspects of neighborhood-based efforts to improve the well-being of individuals, families, and the community as a whole. Speakers were brought in, and a wide variety of topics related to neighborhood and community development were discussed.

After considerable planning and consultation with people experienced in neighborhood and community development, a new project, Community Consultation Services, was also proposed and approved. The purpose of this initiative is to assist citizen groups and community organizations to work effectively together in planning and taking action to improve the quality of community life, or to

---

1. Copies of the Funders' Guide Manual may be purchased by ordering from: Funders' Guide Manual, Community Care Resources, Wilder Foundation, 919 Lafond Ave., St. Paul, MN 55104.

tackle a particular problem or issue in a neighborhood. Under the leadership of a CCR staff person and with funding from several area foundations and the United Way, consultation has been provided to a broadly representative group called Neighbors Acting Together (NAT) in an inner city neighborhood of St. Paul. Activities include a neighborhood needs assessment conducted by volunteers assisted by Wilder Research Center staff, followed by community forums to discuss results of the needs assessment. The forum-style discussions aim to assist residents to identify strengths and visions of the neighborhood, and to form task groups to act on particular objectives.

Another new initiative, the Family Wellness Project, has been undertaken to help disseminate findings from research on characteristics of healthy families. More and more is being learned about the attributes, activities and skills that contribute to personal and family wellness, including communication, appreciation, time together, family routines and rituals, and community involvement. What is missing in many cases is not the aspirations but the tools or skills for families to activate and build on their strengths. The Family Wellness project at Wilder seeks to address that void in three ways. First, a demonstration project is being conducted in the city of St. Paul through which community organizations will develop plans and programs supportive of personal and family wellness for their constituencies and in their communities. Locations are being chosen which will include persons who are from households of different income levels, educational backgrounds, and family structures (including inner-city congregations made up primarily of American Indians and Hmong refugees and one suburban Protestant church). Second, the project is providing leadership by conducting forty to fifty workshops and training experiences for professionals in Minnesota and throughout the country to assist in integrating family wellness information into professional practice and in leading family wellness events. And third, the project is negotiating for a corporate partnership to produce and distribute booklets and other materials related to family wellness, both locally and nationally.

Finally, within a Wilder program which provides treatment services for men and women involved in domestic violence (Community Assistance Program), a preventive effort was begun for the children of adults receiving treatment services. Time-limited groups have been initiated which provide the children opportunities to learn about violence and anger, to identify their own feelings resulting from their exposure to violence in their families, to share common experiences with other children and to learn alternative ways to handle such feelings and experiences. Originally begun as part of the Prevention Planning Project, these groups now operate as a routine part of Community Assistance Program services.

As time and resources permit, other new initiatives may be developed. Two staff members have been compiling information on the use of mass media approaches for the delivery of preventive mental health messages, and a concept paper has been developed on the topic of strengthening marriages by assisting in the development and programming of a local chapter of the Association for Couples in Marriage Enrichment, a mutual-help organization dedicated to strengthening marriages through experiential education and couples support groups.

Assisting Others' Prevention Initiatives

Early in the Prevention Planning Project, an effort was made to identify ways team members could respond to the initiatives of other organizations with assistance in developing, operating or evaluating prevention programming. Because of the previous involvement of Community Care Resources with several other organizations interested in prevention, two opportunities presented themselves quickly. One project involved providing training and evaluation services to Lao Family Community, a mutual assistance association serving Southeast Asian refugees in the Twin Cities area, as they implemented a youth project aimed at improved educational, vocational, family, and life planning on the part of refugee youth. The costs of the training and evaluation provided by Wilder staff were fully reimbursed since they were written into Lao Family Community's original contract for the targeted refugee assistance funding which supported the whole project.

A second project was to evaluate a mass media campaign sponsored by the Minnesota Committee for the Prevention of Child Abuse. A pre-test statewide survey was designed and administered, but the organization was unfortunately unable to complete the mass media campaign, so the evaluation could not be conducted.

As Prevention Planning Team members have learned more about prevention developments in other states, and have increased their contacts with key people in Minnesota and across the country, it has become more and more apparent that significant progress in improving the extent and effectiveness of prevention efforts requires collaborative planning and policy development at the state level, as well as increased grassroots collaborative, inter-organizational cooperation. In order to contribute to efforts at the state level, team members have assisted in convening forums and roundtables to bring together key actors, who, in concert with others, could contribute to systematic planning and action efforts. One forum involved convening people from across the education and health systems to consider the topic of enhancing parent education and support services for parents under stress. Another forum included key people from state departments, advocacy organizations, grant-making foundations, religious groups, and self-help groups, and was called to consider factors involved in effective child abuse prevention. The latter group continued meeting regularly, obtained funding, and put on a two-day invitational, state-wide symposium on promoting healthy families and communities, entitled "Facing the Shadow—Creating New Light." Nearly eighty representatives of county Children's Trust Fund Councils from across the state of Minnesota attended this event.

A team member has also volunteered to serve on an Education and Prevention Task Force of the county human services department. In that capacity the team member contributed to writing a statement addressed to the state mental health department, entitled "Statement of Need for a Coordinated Strategy for Prevention in Human Services in Minnesota." Other team members have served on a teen pregnancy prevention planning committee and on an advisory committee for a pilot effort by the State Department of Education to involve businesses, parents, and schools in developing positive youth development activities in local communities.

Several other organizations have recently requested brief consultation or training around prevention programming, planning, and/or evaluation. Through the Community Care Resources Program and the Prevention Planning Team, additional training and consultation around prevention planning and programming will be offered in the future.

CONCLUSION

A variety of activities have been initiated at the Wilder Foundation to increase awareness and promote the development of effective prevention programming. Some of these could readily be done by personnel in any nonprofit mental health organization if given approval by its administration and board. Others are more likely to be limited to an organization with research capacity and/or adequate financial support for substantial planning and development efforts.

An interdisciplinary team effort was found to be quite valuable, although very time-consuming, for stimulating and guiding the information gathering, conceptualizing, networking and planning required for successful project implementation.

The intention of Wilder's Prevention Planning Team to serve as a prevention resource and to involve direct service professionals in prevention activity was successful to some extent but had to be scaled down as prevention team members attended to the demands of high priority projects. Perhaps even more limitation on the breadth of activities considered and attempted would have strengthened a smaller number of activities. However, the breadth of conceptual explorations by the prevention team did help prepare them to be more effective consultants and resource persons when called upon by funders and other community organizations and agencies.

The efforts of the Wilder Foundation have thus far been well-received in the community. Collaborative relationships have worked very well for the most part, and have been critical to the success of several projects. Extensive and careful planning and nurturing of these relationships has paid dividends, not only in effective project work and involvement of more people and organizations in prevention activity, but also in numerous spin-off effects such as increased referrals and cooperation among different participating agencies outside of their prevention project activities.

REFERENCE

Amherst H. Wilder Foundation. (1984). *Key findings and implications: A survey of 19-34 year olds. In Ramsey County* Office of Research and Statistics, Report #8 January, 1984.

Divorce Workshops: Community Education for a High Risk Population

John Kalafat
St. Clares-Riverside Medical Center

Maureen Underwood
New Jersey Division of Mental Health & Hospitals

Nancy Fiedler
Rutgers Medical School

William D. Neigher
St. Clares-Riverside Medical Center

SUMMARY. The high incidence and prevalence of divorce, as well as its stressful nature, make the divorced and separated population an important target for community preventive intervention programs. A collaboration between a CMHC and a local chapter of Parents Without Partners (PWP) resulted in *Making It!* a series of ten 2.5 hour multimedia educational workshops addressing the impacts of divorce. The series averaged over 100 participants per workshop, and standard epidemiological measures on a subsample of attendees indicated that they were significantly distressed compared to the normative population. Aside from high attendance, and positive participant feedback, other outcomes of this community intervention included the provisions of a variety of additional requested educational programs for divorced persons and community gatekeepers, referrals to the sponsoring CMHC; increased member-

---

Reprints may be obtained from John Kalafat, Department of Education, St. Clares-Riverside Medical Center, Pocono Road, Denville, NJ 07834.

ship and a national award for the PWP Chapter, and the publication of a *Making It!* manual for community educators. While this program has proven to be viable, research needs to be done on its specific impact on participants.

The high incidence and prevalence of divorce as well as the extremely stressful nature of this event have by now been well-documented (Kelly, 1982; Kitson & Raschke, 1981; Kolevzon & Gottlieb, 1983). Morbidity and mortality rates as a function of marital status consistently show that compared to the general population, divorced persons represent a significantly at risk population in terms of a wide variety of physical and psychological disorders, including clinical depression, suicide, homicide, alcoholism and admission to inpatient and outpatient psychiatric facilities (Bloom, Asher, & White, 1978; Levinger, 1976). Bloom, Asher and White (1978) conclude their review of the impact of divorce by stating that the frequency and severity of marital disruption render it "an irresistible candidate for preventive intervention programs that are well thought out, economically feasible, and subject to careful evaluation" (p. 888).

This recommendation is based upon a paradigm for primary prevention described by Bloom (1979). This paradigm assumes that we are all variously vulnerable to stressful life events with which almost any disease or disability may be associated (Dohrenwend & Dohrenwend, 1974). This represents a shift in attention from long-standing predisposing factors in psychopathology to far more recent precipitating factors. On the basis of this paradigm, preventive intervention programs can be organized around facilitating mastery or reducing the incidence of particular stressful life events. According to Bloom's (1979) analysis, "there is every reason to believe that preventive intervention services linked to stressful life events can be enormously effective, particularly when we set about to build on what is already known about crisis theory and crisis intervention" (p. 184). In such cases, the debilitating response, rather than the stressful event, is the preventive target.

Crisis intervention approaches have long consisted of the provision of structure, understanding, information and predictions to individuals caught up in overwhelming, disorienting experiences (Caplan, 1964; Mitchell & Resnik, 1981). Bloom's (1979) further analysis of the literature on (1) the trait of *competence*, consisting of effective coping strategies and a sense of control (Iscoe, 1974; Ryan, 1971), (2) the effects of rapid social *change* (Cassel, 1973) and, (3) the mediating effects of being a part of a *network* of reciprocal relationships that provide confidants feedback and encouragement (Cobb, 1976; Leavy, 1983; Lynch, 1977; Sarason, 1980) indicates that effective programs must address these particular issues. In general then, what is called for are preventive intervention programs that can facilitate mastery of the multiple stresses experienced by large numbers of divorced and separated persons in any given community. Such programs should draw upon and enhance the mutual support capacities of this population.

The field of mental health education appears to include a number of factors necessary to provide an effective response to the needs of the divorced population. The aim of mental health education is to "promote positive mental health by helping people acquire knowledge, attitudes and behavior patterns that will foster and maintain their mental well-being" (National Institute of Mental Health, 1966, p. 4). The targets of mental health education, to be reached by mass media and group education approaches, include the general public, at-risk groups and community caregivers (Adelson & Lurie, 1982; McMillen & Williams, 1977). The strengths of this approach include the fact that it affects large populations, does not require a client or patient status and builds on competencies rather than focusing on pathology (Williams, 1979). After an extensive review of mental health education, Bloom (1984) concluded that, "for psychological disorders, no approach to health maintenance for disease management holds more promise than mental health education" (p. 350).

With the dramatic increase of divorce in the early 70s it became clear to a number of practitioners that traditional clinical approaches which emphasize pathology and a dyadic "waiting" mode were insufficient for addressing this societal problem (Glidewell, 1971; Nichols, 1977; Shelton & Nix, 1979). As early as 1975, the literature contains descriptions of educational approaches to divorce intervention. The format employed was small lecture-discussion groups variously titled "Seminars for the Separated" (Weiss,

1975), "Adjustment to Divorce" (Nichols, 1977) or "Divorce and Personal Growth Seminars" (Fisher, 1978).

The goals of these groups have generally been to provide information about the divorcing process and to deal with the psychological reaction to disruption; to provide assistance and advice around practical issues such as child rearing, finance, employment and legal issues; and to furnish emotional support derived mainly from others who have undergone or are undergoing a similar experience (Bloom, Asher, & White, 1978). The groups have been time-limited, ranging in length from ten sessions (Fisher, 1978) to a single four-hour workshop (Young, 1978) with the majority clustering around four to eight sessions (Bonkowski & Wanner-Westly, 1979; Nichols, 1977; Shelton & Nix, 1979; Weiss, 1985). The number of participants tended to be limited to eight to ten to maximize opportunities for interaction.

Evaluations of two such educational programs provide encouraging evidence as to their utility. Young (1978) evaluated a four-hour divorce workshop through pre, post and three-month follow-up participant reports of divorce-related concerns and post and three-month follow-up reports of the effects of the workshop. Both provided evidence of the positive impact of the workshop. Bloom, Hodges and Caldwell (1982) evaluated a six-month program which made paraprofessional counselors available on individual and group bases to cohorts of divorced persons. Specific subject-matter study groups were also available to participants. Participant feedback was positive and changes on pre, post and six-month follow-up measures of neuresthenia and anxiety showed significant positive changes not found in a comparison group.

Both Young and Bloom and his associates identified shortcomings of their programs and made suggestions for improvements. Both cited the fact that divorce is a long process with different issues at different stages and thus programs should cover a longer period of time and address such issues. Neither program addressed significantly large numbers of people, and Bloom cited the need to maintain sufficient attendance to provide the positive effects of group interaction.

Both programs depended on contact with professionals or trained paraprofessional caregivers as opposed to being programs embedded in the community that could establish and maintain an ongoing community support system.

Bloom (1984) indicated that programs involving active participation tend to be more successful. This, plus the focus of educational groups on emotional and practical problems experienced by divorcing persons, follows the classic components of effective adult education identified by Knowles (1973). Based on over thirty years of research and experience in the ways adults learn, Knowles recommended that educational programs be centered on problems currently experienced by participants rather than on abstract content, draw upon and affirm participants' experiences, and actively involve them in the process. Other educational data (e.g., Sredl & Rothwell, 1987) indicate that programs should contain a mix of media and formats for maximum retention.

The application of these recommendations will next be described in a divorce education program for the authors' county.

NEEDS ASSESSMENT AND PLANNING

The county in which the program was offered mirrored the national rising trend in divorces. Between 1970 and 1980, the percent of divorced and separated rose from 3.25% to 5.95% while the percent married dropped from 66.9% to 60.9%. During the eighteen-month period of the project, 3,860 divorces were granted in the county, ranking it third among the 21 counties in the state.

The program originated with a request for educational services by officers of the local chapter of Parents Without Partners (PWP). PWP is a nationally organized self-help group that was well established in the state with chapters in each county. The PWP charter calls for the provision of educational programming and such a request was consistent with the public health orientation of the Community Systems Division (CSD) of St. Clares-Riverside Medical Center Community Mental Health Center. Based on the initial meetings with PWP officers, it was decided that a series of educational workshops would be co-sponsored by PWP and the CSD.

The CSD agreed to conduct a needs assessment with PWP members, develop with PWP officers a set of educational workshops and make a "package" of the workshops available to the local and regional PWP organization. PWP would assist in the planning and delivery of the workshops, provide all publicity through local newspapers, radio spots and their monthly newsletter and arrange for a meeting site in the community to minimize the stigma that often accompanies mental-health sponsored programming (Guerney & Jordan, 1979). The joint planning and sponsorship of the workshops by PWP, and the arrangement whereby PWP staff would gradually phase-in as presentors and workshop manuals would be made available to local and regional PWP officers, were attempts to ensure that this community education would be ensconced as an ongoing *community* support service as recommended by Bloom, Hodges and Caldwell (1982).

In addition to a thorough literature search (which went beyond the professional literature to include popular books on divorce) and discussions with PWP officers acting as key informants, the needs assessment and planning was carried out by attendance by CSD staff at several "coffee and conversation" meetings at the homes of PWP members, and the collection at a PWP social function of 80 open-ended surveys of major needs and issues of divorcing/divorced persons. The meetings and surveys both tapped members at the local county PWP chapter which was the target group for the intervention.

The workshop series then, was grounded in current knowledge about the divorce process, mental health education, crisis intervention and adult learning. It was shaped by the feedback from PWP members and officers. PWP officers chose the title *Making It!* for the series because of their desire for an upbeat, coping theme.

MAKING IT! *SERIES*

Crisis literature (cf. Caplan, 1964) plus the literature on competence and social networks (cf. Bloom, 1979) call for a program that provides *structure* and *understanding* of a complex and overwhelming process as well as *coping strategies* and the mediating effects of a *social network.* The PWP officers and members echoed these needs in their call for information about and ways to deal with the impacts of divorce and the opportunity to share this educational process with others in a similar situation.

These needs were translated into the goals and objectives for the workshops: (a) practical information that would provide structure and understanding concerning the impacts of divorce as well as about effective coping strategies; and (b) the support and hope derived from meeting and sharing experiences and problem solving with others in similar circumstances. The objectives of the series were:

1. to organize the crises of divorce into a recognizable process;
2. to normalize the divorcing experience within a supportive context; and
3. to reinforce the competencies participants already possessed to aid them in the resolution of problems precipitated by separation and divorce.

Paul Bohannan's (1971) stations of divorce seemed to capture the many impacts of divorce and thus served as the organizing framework for the first time workshops. The stations are:

1. Emotional divorce – begins when the spouses withhold emotional investment in the relationship, usually occurs before the separation for at least one partner.
2. Legal divorce – occurs when the final decree is handed down by the judge.
3. Economic divorce – involves dividing the possessions, setting up separate households and budgets.
4. Coparental divorce – decisions about custody and separation of mothering and fathering roles.
5. Community divorce – responding to reactions of family and friends and loosening bonds with some old friends and beginning new friendships.
6. Psychic divorce – establishing a new identity as a single individual separate from the spouse.

These were translated into workshops which emphasized the issues captured in the needs assessment. The first five workshops which were approved by the PWP officers were:

1. The Impact of Divorce, Part I – The Adult
2. The Community Divorce – Reactions of Family and Friends
3. The Impact of Divorce, Part II – The Child
4. Especially for Men; Especially for Women
5. The Challenge of Being Single

The workshops were 2.5 hours long and were offered bi-weekly over a three-month period. All programs were multi-media, utilizing either videotapes, or slides, in addition to lecturettes, role plays, handouts and structured group interaction. Table 1 depicts the typical workshop format. The role plays involved the consultants, PWP officers and audience members. The role plays demonstrated typical dilemmas encountered by the divorcing individual as identified in the needs assessment. In this way, the workshops followed Knowles' recommendations for learning related to participants current problems, involving active participation and acknowledging learners' experiences. The small groups segment was purposely task-oriented and generally focused around the discussion and resolution of commonly experienced problems while leaving sufficient time for spontaneous interaction among participants. It was felt that minimal structuring would limit the obsessional review which often monopolizes group discussions, albeit a necessary component in personal resolution of divorce (Weiss, 1975). The small group discussion was designed to provide the competence-enhancing coping

TABLE 1

Typical Divorce Workshop Format

Introduction of Topic and Speakers	5 minutes
Lecturette with audio/visual aids and handouts	15 minutes
Live or videotape demonstration of points	15 minutes
Break	15 minutes
Audience Participation: Roleplay or Exercise	20-40 minutes
Small Group Discussion: Structured Context provided	30-40 minutes
Report back to large group (optional)	0-10 minutes
Feedback Forms and Research Forms	20 minutes

strategies and network of feedback and encouragement. The participants were the "experts" while the consultants were facilitators.

This initial workshop series focused on the many impacts of the divorce process per se. A logical sequel to this series consisted of workshops that addressed the ongoing issues that occupy newly single adults. Feedback obtained from participants in the initial series confirmed that they wished us to turn our attention to such post-impact issues.

A second five-session series which was offered monthly with essentially the same format as the first was then developed. The topics were derived from the aforementioned participant feedback and from the review of the divorce literature. These topics included:

1. Learning to Love Again
2. You and Your Kids: Approaches to Parenting
3. Your Relationship with your Ex-Spouse – Friend or Enemy? Custody Issues and Other Negotiations
4. Sexuality and the Single Parent
5. Package Deals: New Spouses, Old Children.

While participants were somewhat heterogeneous as to the stages of the divorce process, the sequencing from initial impact to ongoing issues appeared to be most responsive to participants' needs.

Demographic data were collected at two of the workshops (n = 45 & 55; approximately 50% return rate). Seventy percent of the participants were female; all were white with a mean age of 41 years. Slightly more than 30% had college degrees and the mean income was $30,000 for males and $15,600 for females. The post-divorce income level for females represented a 50% drop from their reported income while married, while men reported an average post divorce income of approximately $3,500 higher than while married. Whether support payments were included in male or female incomes is not known. The participants, thus, were white, middle-aged, educated individuals. As such, they were fairly representative of the county as a whole. The county demographics were based on the 1980 census and indicate that the county was 95% white; 29% of those over 25 years old had completed college; and that the mean income was $33,469 for white households. Participants had been married for an average of 16 years (range: 3-26) and divorced for an average of 1.6 years (range: 3 months-4 years).

PROCESS EVALUATION

Community Response

The response to the first series of workshops indicated that they were addressing a widely felt need. The attendance averaged slightly more than 100 per workshop. The lone exception was the final workshop on remarriage which may have been premature for this audience. This was the only workshop for which attendance dropped significantly below 100 (n = 55-60). An alternate account for this attendance drop might be the year-end waning of enthusiasm, which was certainly felt by the leaders. The total attendance, then, was approximately 1,100. Based upon attendance sheets, the unduplicated attendance was approximately 750.

Participant Feedback

Open-ended feedback forms were passed out at each workshop. They consisted of six questions: (1) What did you expect to get out of coming tonight? (2) What part of tonight's program was most helpful to you? (3) What did you like the least? (4) If you could attend more meetings, what would you like them to cover? (5) Would you please rate the overall quality of the workshop (Excellent, Very Good, Good, Fair, Poor). An average of 45 forms were collected at each workshop.

A review of the contents of the forms revealed a consistent set of expectations including meeting others in the same situation; sharing experiences with others; obtaining general information; learning specific strategies for coping and gaining insight into oneself, others and the divorce process; and receiving emotional support (also described as courage, resolve, hope, confirmation, less guilt). It is interesting to note that these responses are quite consistent with those of participants in a variety of other self-help groups (Knight et al., 1980; Levy, 1979). As a nationally organized self-help group, with an educational charter, PWP appeared to be meeting some generic member needs by brokering with human service providers (each of whom, happened to share the condition with the members). This is, then, a good example of a collaboration between human service providers and a self-help group which did not attenuate the autonomy of the group. By phasing in PWP officers and providing the detailed manual, the professionals also did not promote continued dependency on the consultants to meet these needs.

The specific parts of the workshop that were rated most helpful included the expertise of the leaders, normalization, explanation of the stages and process of divorce, and open discussion about feelings and coping techniques. The structured group discussions were cited as helpful more often than the lectures, media, roleplays or written materials, again confirming the value of mutual support for participants.

Few negative reactions were listed. The major complaint was the large size of the discussion groups (there were only enough leaders for five 'small' groups which had over 20 members when attendance was over 100). A moderate amount of negative feedback was also received on a slide presentation on family stereotypes and values that proved too evocative for separated and divorced persons. Finally, participants expressed the desire for more "how to" information in two different categories, (1) feelings – how to deal with rejection, hostility, guilt, anxiety; and (2) pragmatics – how to date, meet people, answer children's questions, and so forth.

This feedback was not only helpful for evaluating these workshops but also for planning further workshops, including a second segment of this series. Participants' reported expectations were quite similar to the leaders' goals and objectives for this series as well as for the other workshops reported in the literature. The reported benefits confirmed the leaders' hopes for the workshops – particularly in the areas of normalization, explanation and the provision of emotional support and hope.

Additional feedback was obtained from participants in a slightly revised 8 session *Making It!* series given in the year following the first *Making It!* series. These participants were very similar to these on the first series in terms of age, sex, race, length of marriage and length of time divorced. Responses were obtained from all the participants (n = 45) at the final workshop. These responses are summarized in Table 2. The responses appear to be a face-valid esti-

TABLE 2

Impact of Divorce Workshops: Participants' Response

Did participation in the workshops: (Please check one)

	Yes	No	Not Applicable
Influence your attitude about divorce	50%	37%	13%
Influence your attitude toward your ex-spouse	40%	57%	3%
Help in the legal aspects of the divorce process	16%	58%	26%
Help you deal with the reactions of family and friends to your divorce	58%	32%	10%
Help you deal with your emotional reactions to the divorce (grief, anger)	67%	21%	12%
Help you explain the divorce to your child(ren)	42%	29%	29%
Help you deal with your child's emotional reaction to the divorce	63%	20%	17%
Influence your feelings about being single again	71%	23%	6%
Clarify religious considerations about divorce	12%	62%	27%
Give you methods or techniques to help you deal with being single again	80%	17%	3%
Change your view about the opposite sex	32%	52%	16%
Help you adjust to your custody arrangement	33%	30%	37%

mate of the workshops' effects. That is, areas that were addressed very briefly (i.e., legal aspects) or not at all (i.e., religious considerations) were rated by very few respondents. On the other hand, those areas rated by the most respondents (i.e., emotional reactions, child's reactions, feelings about being single and techniques for being single) were covered most thoroughly in the series.

It was hoped that the workshops would have a greater impact on participants' attitudes toward their ex-spouses and the opposite sex. However, one of the clearest lessons from this extensive contact with divorced persons has been that negative feelings in these areas are extraordinarily recalcitrant. A crisis/educational approach may not be effective for dealing with more "clinical" issues that appear to be centered around attachment (Weiss, 1975) and narcissistic injury (Rice, 1977).

This, again, is an argument for the provision of preventive educational programs by comprehensive community based human services or by consultants who have close ties to such services. That is, a number of issues can be raised in such large scale educational workshops that may require a more extensive or intensive follow-up with some participants.

One of the effects of such educational outreaches to the community by a Community Mental Health Center is an increase in the psychological accessibility, defined as normalization or lack of stigma associated with use of the agency and its secondary and tertiary services, to the target population. In these workshops, the presentors were representatives of the CMHC, and as participants became more familiar and impressed with them, they were more likely to avail themselves of the CMHC's traditional clinical services. As will be detailed later, this was one of the outcomes of this series.

It should be noted that the workshop series is a preventive educational intervention according to Bloom's (1979) paradigm. As such, the goal of the series is the prevention or attenuation of a debilitating response to a stressful life event, and not "case finding" for the sponsoring community mental health center. However, such community education interventions invariably have such "ripple" effects on other parts of the service system. A comprehensive agency or service network's response to clients who might not otherwise have availed themselves of its services demonstrates the close linkage, if not slight blurring, among primary, secondary and tertiary interventions.

EPIDEMIOLOGICAL STRESS DATA

The basic goal of the series was to provide educational and supportive services to a greater number of at-risk individuals than had heretofore been reached through small-group or clinical approaches. While a large number of separated and divorced individuals attended the workshops, the question may be raised as to whether this series reached a significantly at-risk population.

One way of assessing this is to ascertain how distressed workshop participants were compared to individuals presenting themselves to the CMHC for services and to a sample of the general population. To answer these questions, standard epidemiological measures were selected with established reliability and validity and for which scores on a normative population were available.

The measures used were the Brief Symptom Inventory (BSI) which is a shorter version of the Symptom Checklist-90 (SCL-90) developed by Derogatis (1977); and the Center for Epidemiology Studies Depression Scale (CES-D) developed by CES at the National Institute for Mental Health (Radloff, 1977).

Each scale is a self report symptom inventory that has community norms and reliability and validity data. Respondents were asked to indicate how they felt during the past seven days.

The BSI is a 53 item scale with each item rated on the same five point scale as the SCL-40 and the same nine symptom dimensions and their global scales. Since the BSI symptom scales correlate in the 92-99 range with the SCL-90, the same reliability and validity estimates for the SCL-90 apply to the BSI.

The CES-D scale is a 20 item scale with each item rated on a 4 point scale. It has proven reliability and validity and extensive normative data (Radloff, 1977).

These measures were administered to these groups:

1. A sample of *Making It!* participants (BSI n = 35; CES-D n = 19). This sample was obtained by handing out measures to the first 45 participants at a workshop and collecting them the following week. These respondents were demographically similar to the other samples of workshop participants and did not significantly differ from them in terms of average length of marriage or divorce. With this data collection procedure and the return rate, particularly for the CES-D, we cannot rule out the possibility that this group might be unrepresentative of the overall workshop participants in terms of their level of distress.
2. A sample of adults presenting themselves for outpatient clini-

cal services at the CMHC serving the same community for which the workshop was offered (BSI n = 37; CES-D n = 39). This sample was obtained by requesting successive clients during the time the workshops were offered to complete the measures until 40 measures were obtained. The final n was due to missing data or incorrectly completed forms. This sample was similar to the PWP sample in sex, education and race, but was significantly younger (35.9-40.5) and had less children (1.79-2.46); of course, they differed in terms of marital status in that 8% of them were separated or divorced.

A third comparison group was afforded by the normative population data on the two measures.

Results indicated that the PWP group and the CMHC group were significantly more distressed than the nonpatient normative group on the BSI scales of obsession-compulsive, interpersonal sensitivity, depression, anxiety, hostility, paranoia, psychoticism, global severity index, and positive symptom index and on the CES-D. No significant differences were found between the PWP and the CMHC samples. Also, data were available for a formerly married subsample of the CES-D normative sample, and both the PWP and CMHC were significantly more distressed than formerly married normative sample group.

Thus, there is some evidence that workshop participants may have been equally as distressed as CMHC clients and that both were more distressed than nonpatient community members, including divorced community members. This community education program, then, appeared to achieve its goal of reaching a significantly distressed population.

ADDITIONAL PROGRAM IMPACT

As previously noted, an educational outreach program such as this tends to have a ripple effect on various components of the community system in which it is implemented. The major identified effects were on the two organizations that co-sponsored the series.

PWP

The local chapter of PWP reported a considerable increase in membership during the course of the series and won a community service award from the national PWP organization for their sponsorship and involvement in the program. They co-sponsored a condensed eight session repeat of the program the following year. (We were revising two of the workshops based on our experience and as part of our preparation of the manual.) This series gave PWP officers an opportunity to assume the leadership of the workshops with the consultants assisting. This process was invaluable in the preparation of a manual that would be used by PWP officers and community gatekeepers as well as professional consultants. Attendance at these workshops averaged 55 per session, which is still quite high for such programs.

CMHC

A question was added to the participant evaluation form for the last session of the original series that asked participants if they had sought any form of counseling since their attendance at the workshop and 12.5% indicated that they had come to the sponsoring CMHC. Based on the total unduplicated attendance of approximately 750, we can reliably estimate that the series may have generated at least 94 direct referrals to the CMHC. This figure does not include the friends and family members that the participants referred to the CMHC as a result of their involvement in the workshops. Based on group leaders' contacts with participants and CMHC staff, we estimate that this figure may represent another 90 or more persons. These data must, of course, be qualified by the fact that we cannot be sure how many of these individuals would have come to the community mental health center in the absence of the workshops.

Related follow-up, fee-generating programs were provided at the CMHC, including a single parents discussion group, a working parents workshop and discussion groups for men's issues. Local newspaper coverage and presentations at regional and national conferences resulted in numerous additional workshops and consults to a wide variety of community agencies. Also, as originally contracted, a detailed workshop manual and accompanying videotape was developed by the CMHC and made available to PWP. The CMHC sold over 300 copies of the manual through word of mouth, and a revised version has been published for national distribution (Underwood and Kalafat, 1988).

CONCLUSION

At this point, we have only indirect evidence of the cost effectiveness of this program. There is evidence for the efficacy of a similar program (Bloom, Hodges, & Caldwell, 1982) for divorced and separated persons. The present program incorporated the recommendations for improved efficacy made by those authors and should now be assessed as to its impact on participants. This could be done by presenting another *Making It!* series and assessing the distress levels of participants and a demographically matched group of divorced persons prior to and after the workshops.

In regard to the cost of the program, it should be noted that the major cost to the CMHC was the staff time involved in the development of the series. PWP bore the cost of the publicity, site and refreshments; shared the cost of materials; and contributed staff time to the implementation and development of the program. It appears that if a program is truly meeting an acknowledged community need, the community (e.g., a self-help organization, corporation, school system) will assist in paying for it.

The CMHC staff time devoted to the development of the original series was quite high. The preparation ratio for at least the first five workshops is estimated to be as high as 30 hours of preparation per hour of presentation. As the consultants gained familiarity with the issues and resources in the area of divorce, this rate was reduced. As the program was disseminated and other related community consultations and educational programs were provided, the return on the time investment became increasingly favorable.

Marital disruption is clearly a complex process that unfolds over time. It is of such high incidence that some argue that it is best conceived of as a normative life transition (Ahrons, 1980). In light of the high incidence and prevalence of marital disruption and its stressful sequelae, it would appear that extended, large-scale intervention programs can be an important component of comprehensive care for high risk populations. It is felt that this program represents an apparently successful collaborative venture between a CMHC and a community self-help organization to develop, field-test and package a program that appears to respond to the needs of this population and has proven to be of sustained interest.

REFERENCES

Adelson, D., & Lurie, L. (1972). Mental health education: Research and practice. In S.E. Golan & C. Eisdorfer (Eds.), *Handbook of community mental health*. New York: Appleton-Century-Crofts.

Ahrons, C. R. (1980). Divorce: A crisis of family transition and change. *Family Relations*, *24*, 533-540.

Bloom, B. L. (1979). Prevention of mental disorders: Recent advances in theory and practice. *Community Mental Health Journal*, *3*, 179-181.

Bloom, B. L. (1984). *Community mental health: A general introduction*. Monterey, CA: Brooks/Cole.

Bloom, B. L., Asher, S. J., & White, S. W. (1978). Marital disruption as a stressor: A review and analysis. *Psychological Bulletin*, *85*, 867-894.

Bloom, B. L., Hodges, W. F., & Caldwell, R.A. (1982). A preventive intervention program for the newly separated: Initial evaluation. *American Journal of Community Psychology*, *10*, 251-264.

Bohannan, P. (1971). *Divorce and after*. Garden City, NY: Doubleday & Co.

Bonkowski, S. W., & Wanner-Westly, B. (1979). The divorce group: A new treatment modality. *Social Casework*, *9*, 552-557.

Caplan, G. (1964). *Principles of preventive psychiatry*. New York: Basic Books.

Cassel, J. (1973). The relation of the urban environment to health: Implications for prevention. *Mount Sinai Journal of Medicine*, *40*, 539-550.

Cobb, S. (1976). Social support as a moderator of life stress. *Psychosomatic Medicine*, *38*, 300-314.

Derogatis, L. (1977). *SCL-90 Revised Version Manual I.* Baltimore: Johns Hopkins University School of Medicine.

Dohrenwend, B. S., & Dohrenwend, B. P. (Eds.). (1974). *Stressful life events: Their nature and effects*. New York: Wiley.

Fisher, B. (1978). *When your relationship ends*. Boulder, CO: Family Relations Learning Center.

Glidewell, J.C. (1971). Priorities for psychologists in community mental health. In Division 27, American Psychological Association, Task Force on Community Mental Health, *Issues in community psychology and preventive mental health*. New York: Behavioral Publications.

Guerney, L., & Jordan, L. (1979). Children of divorce: A community support group. *Journal of Divorce*, *3*, 282-292.

Iscoe, I. (1974). Psychology and the competent community. *American Psychologist*, *29*, 607-623.

Kelly, J. (1982). Divorce: The adult perspective. In B. Wolman & G. Stricker (Eds.), *Handbook of Developmental Psychology*. New York: Prentice-Hall.

Kitson, F. C., & Raschke, H. J. (1981). Divorce research: What we know; what we need to know. *Journal of Divorce*, *4*, 1-38.

Knight, B., Wollert, R. W., Levy, L. H., Frame, C. L., & Padgett, V. P. (1980). Self-help groups: The members' perspective. *American Journal of Community Psychology*, *1*, 53-66.

Knowles, M. (1973). *The adult learner: A neglected species*. Houston, TX: Gulf Publishing.

Kolevzon, M. S., & Gottlieb, S. J. (1982). The impact of divorce: A multivariate study. *Journal of Divorce*, *2*, 19-98.

Leavy, R. L. (1983). Social support and psychological disorder: A review. *Journal of Community Psychology*, *1*, 3-21.

Levinger, G. (1976). A social psychological perspective on marital dissolution. *Journal of Social Issues*, *32*, 21-48.

Levy, L.H. (1979). Processes and activities in groups. In M.A. Lieberman, L.D. Borman, and Associates (Eds.), *Self-help groups for coping with crisis*. San Francisco: Jossey-Bass.

Lynch, J.J. (1976). *The broken heart*. New York: Basic Books.

National Institution of Mental Health. (1966). *Consultation and education*. US-PHS Pub. No. 1478. Washington, DC: U.S. Government Printing Office.

Nichols, W. C. (1977). Divorce and remarriage education. *Journal of Divorce*, *2*, 153-159.

Radloff, L.S. (1977) The CES-D scale: A self report depression scale for research in the general population. *Applied Psychological Measurement,* 1, 385-401.

Rice, D. G. (1977). Psychotherapeutic treatment of narcissistic injury in marital separation and divorce. *Journal of Divorce*, *2*, 119-128.

Ryan, W. (1971). *Blaming the victim*. New York: Random House.

Sarason, I. G. (1980). Life stress, self-preoccupation and social supports. In I. G. Sarason & C.D. Spielburger (Eds.), *Stress and Anxiety* (Vol. 7). Washington: Halsted.

Shelton, S. C., & Nix, C. (May 1979). Development of a divorce adjustment group program in a social service agency. *Social Casework*, 309-311.

Smith, W. G. (1971). Critical Life-events and prevention strategies in mental health. *Archives of General Psychiatry*, *25*, 102-109.

Sredl, H.J., & Rothwell, W.J. (1987). *The ASTD reference guide to professional training roles and competencies, Vol II.* Amherst, Mass.: HRD Press Inc.

Underwood, M. M., & Kalafat, J. (1988) *Making it! A manual for community education on divorce and separation*. Dubuque, Iowa: Kendall/Hunt Publishing Company

Weiss, R. S. (1975). *Marital separation*. New York: Basic Books.

Williams, R.T. (1979). *Mental health education: The untapped resource*. Unpublished paper, University of Wisconsin Extension.

Young, D. (1978). The divorce experience: A consumer evaluation. *Journal of Divorce*, *2*, 37-47.

Maximizing the Potential for Community Self-Help Through Clearinghouse Approaches

Edward J. Madara
St. Clares-Riverside Medical Center

SUMMARY. An overview of self-help groups is provided and their relationship to prevention and mental health is discussed. It is suggested that mental health centers would benefit from the increased use and support of groups, and that self-help clearinghouse approaches may be of special benefit. The development of an integrated and multidisciplinary self-help clearinghouse approach to increasing the awareness, utilization, and development of mutual aid self-help groups in the community, with examples of strategies and accomplishments, is described. Principles and concepts important to professionals working with groups are proposed. Trends in the development of health related groups and computer conferencing initiatives are discussed.

There is an analogy that compares the traditional mental health system to an ambulance service laboriously operating at the bottom of a cliff. People are continuously falling from the top of the cliff above to receive triage and treatment below. With services focused upon the crises and needs at the bottom, little attention is directed to the top. This continues until one day it is finally observed that an increasing number of survivors have ascended the cliff on their own and, along with others on the edge, are helping each other from falling by linking together, building fences, and educating others to the danger. It is then that those working below begin to realize that

Requests for reprints should be sent to Edward J. Madara, Self-Help Clearinghouse, St. Clares-Riverside Medical Center, Denville, NJ 07834.

much of the effective action that needs to be supported and recognized is actually taking place at the top of the cliff.

It has been a decade since the President's Commission on Mental Health (1978) recommended increased linkage between mental health services and community support networks. Subsequent national recommendations specifically encouraged the development and utilization of self-help groups (Swift, 1979; U.S. Department of Health & Human Services, 1980). Over the years, mental health centers have explored the benefits associated with developing a broad range of member-run mutual help groups (Chutis, 1983; Hess, 1978; Silverman, 1978). Related efforts have led to the development of self-help clearinghouse programs as a primary means to tapping community self-help groups and potential (Borck & Aronowitz, 1982; Borman & Lieberman, 1979; Jeger, Slotnick, & Schure, 1982; Madara, 1985, 1986, 1987; Wollert, 1985; Wollert & Barron, 1983; Wollert & Self-Help Research Team, 1987). Essentially, self-help clearinghouses help people to find and form self-help groups, while also promoting increased awareness of their availability of groups and an understanding of their functions. Of the fifty-three self-help clearinghouses currently serving nearly half the population of the United States, approximately half have been started by mental health service agencies. Many of these self-help clearinghouses demonstrate some of the unique approaches and methods that exist for professionals to better understand and tap self-help group resources and potential in their own local communities.

There are a variety of reasons why increased mental health agency involvement with self-help groups can prove beneficial. In terms of prevention, the self-help modality holds special potential for addressing the mental health needs of at risk populations such as persons facing transitional life crises, persons with addictions, persons with chronic health problems or disabilities; and families of these individuals. With the decline of traditional community social networks, social isolation continues to be a major problem that affects both mental and physical health. This is especially true for those at risk populations who are facing a stressful life change, illness, loss, addiction, or disability. Self-help groups help to prevent psychopathology by serving as new sources of social support that help people deal with these short-term crises and life transitions as well as the long-term disabilities and stresses. Thus, Albee (1982) cited support groups as a key element in his formula for reducing the incidence of mental disorders:

$$\text{incidence} = \frac{\text{organic factors} + \text{stress}}{\text{coping skills} + \text{self esteem} + \text{support groups}}$$

Self-help groups are also uniquely suited to promoting coping skills and self-esteem through the practical experiential knowledge that is shared, the provision of positive role models usually not available in the professional milieu, and the benefits of being able to help others (Riessman, 1965). Groups are also uniquely suited to extend mental health support to unserved portions of the population. By offering assistance in a non-threatening manner, self-help groups attract and assist those who for a variety of reasons would be hesitant or unwilling to use traditional mental health services. Within the groups, such persons can learn from those who have used mental health services and who personally testify to their value, facilitating referrals to those services when there is the need.

To varying degrees, self-help groups serve their general prevention function by enhancing social ties and connections that can serve as a buffer to stress (Katz & Hermalin, 1987), and by promoting the competency of people to cope with stress and adversity (Silverman, 1985) for a full spectrum of life transitions and crises. Silverman additionally points out that many stressful life transitions cannot be prevented, but that mutual help groups may be one of the more powerful modalities for facilitating the learning of coping skills subsequent to stress.

Parents Anonymous is an example of how such learning can be a preventive intervention, as the group helps break the vicious cycle of child abuse by halting parental abuse of children who would otherwise grow up to be abusive parents themselves. An independent national evaluation of Parents Anonymous conducted by Behavior Associates of Tucson, Arizona (cited in Parents Anonymous, 1976) revealed that of the 19% of group members who physically abused their children on a daily basis before joining Parents Anonymous, only 1% reported continuing such abuse immediately after joining the group.

One example of how self-help groups for stressful life crises may help prevent dysfunction can be drawn from the comments of Mental Patient Liberation Movement leader, Judi Chamberlin. Recounting how a miscarriage caused the depression that led to her psychiatric hospitalization (Chamberlin, 1978), she noted that if miscarriage self-help groups, which have become more numerous in later years, had been available to her at that time, she would have in all probability never suffered the tragic hospitalization that she did (personal communication, April 23,1982). While many groups exist to alleviate the stress associated with specific life transitions and losses, it should also be noted that many focus efforts on the prevention of problems and stress in the community: from spinal cord injury groups teaching accident prevention classes to laryngectomy club members speaking before students on the importance of not smoking; or from the successful advocacy efforts of Mothers Against Drunk Driving (MADD) to the work of Parents of Near-Drowners (POND) in promoting improved safety standards for the pool construction industry.

In dealing with rising demand and limited resources, mental health centers can at a minimum identify and use self-help groups to meet the expanding mental health needs of their communities without having to expand their budgets. For caring clinicians with heavy caseloads, who are trying to meet the many and varied needs of their patients, self-help groups can be a welcome adjunct. Groups can meet needs for peer support that staff cannot address, while often providing help and buddy systems at hours that staff are not available. In addition to supplementing treatment services and increasing client satisfaction, the use of groups can improve discharge planning by providing long-term aftercare support that can reduce recidivism. Centers that support self-help can be expected to improve community public relations. In an American Hospital Association survey of ninety-nine hospitals that had relationships with groups, the majority of respondents listed public relations as the primary benefit of their involvement (Giloth, 1981). Groups can also educate professionals to gaps and problems in service delivery, serve as allies in the development of needed programs, social action or funding efforts, and provide new opportunities for collaboration between the self-help and professional communities.

While older self-help groups like Alcoholics Anonymous and Recovery, which were started in the 1930's, are relatively well-known, the hundreds of other self-help groups that have developed over the last fifteen years for a wide variety of other problems are unfamiliar to most in the public and professional communities. One study reported a dramatic increase in the number of persons involved in self-help groups from an estimated 5 million in 1978 to 14 million in 1984 (U.S. Department of Health & Human Services, 1986). An initial study conducted at the New Jersey Clearinghouse (Leventhal, Maton, & Madara, 1988) found that the overall number of self-help groups in New Jersey was growing at a rate of 8.4% annually. In recent years new national groups such as the National Depressive and Manic Depressive Association, Incest Survivors Anonymous, Adult Children of Alcoholics, National Mental Health Consumers Association, and National Association of People with AIDS have experienced rapid growth. Older groups such as the National Alliance for the Mentally Ill, Narcotics Anonymous, Tough Love, and Survivors of Suicide continue to expand the number of their affiliate groups. New national groups continue to appear, such as the Obsessive-Compulsive Disorders Foundation, Agoraphobics in Motion, Anorexia Nervosa & Associated Disorders Inc., and N.O.S.A.D. – the National Organization for Seasonal Affective Disorders.

New Jersey Clearinghouse staff identified four common characteristics that fundamentally define these self-help groups. First and foremost is the dynamic process of mutual help, people helping people, that is basic to self-help groups. Knowledge is pooled, experiences are shared, hopes are reinforced, and efforts are joined as members strive to help one another. Secondly, groups are composed of peers, who share a common problem or stressful life situation, and who therefore provide a powerful "you are not alone" sense of understanding and peer support, often from the very first contact they have with one another. Thirdly, they are voluntary non-profit groups that charge no fees and have only minimal dues if any. Finally, the groups are run by and for their members, that is the locus of control is with the group members rather than with professionals or others outside the group. This last characteristic has crucial implications. It assures that the activities of the group will appropriately address the true felt needs of its members, rather than their needs as perceived by others. It also provides the members with a sense of true ownership, responsibility, and community. Also, control promotes an important sense of ownership, whereby the extent to which members perceive the group as "their group" will determine the amount of investment they make in, and responsibility they take for, making the group succeed.

PROFESSIONAL INVOLVEMENT WITH SELF-HELP

Professionals have served a variety of roles in supporting self-help groups. They have ranged from providing referrals, to being a guest speaker, from serving as a group advisor to making agency space and clerical services available to groups. But probably the most productive role over the long term has been the work of individual professionals to help lay persons to develop new groups. In an early county-wide survey of different types of self-help groups, clearinghouse staff found that approximately one third of the existing groups had been started with the help of a professional. It should be pointed out, however, that many of those groups reporting professional help were individual groups that had no affiliation with a national self-help organization; whereas, those reporting no professional help were usually nationally affiliated and had multiple chapters in each county. By the very nature of their specialty work, professionals are often in a very favorable position to identify, encourage, and link together persons who have the potential to start a mutual help group for a specific mental health problem.

The history of self-help groups illustrates how individual professionals have played major roles in developing several national self-help organizations, e.g., a psychiatrist starting Recovery Inc., a social worker linking clients to form Parents Anonymous, a physician starting Mended Hearts, a clergyman helping to form Compassionate Friends. Other professionals have played a variety of roles in helping to support the development and promotion of self-help groups. Yet, while some professionals have become more aware of the value of self-help groups, few understand the basic principles and benefits of self-determination, mutual help, helper therapy, and empowerment that contribute to the very success and viability of these groups. In a 1983 New Jersey conference on Self-Help and Mental Health, Marie Killilea of Johns Hopkins University School of Hygiene and Public Health stressed an important point in reference to professional–self-help interface in noting that "the first thing that professionals have to learn about self-help groups is that there is something to learn." A major problem that many professionals face is that they are not educated to the number and variety of self-help groups or to their distinctive benefits. Most have yet to discover the roles that they as professionals can play in utilizing, developing and supporting these resources. It would appear that the underlying problem is the fact that the subject of self-help groups is not significantly addressed in graduate training curricula, such as that of social workers (Black & Drachman 1985). Like members of self-help groups, most professionals have had to acquire much of their education about self-help through "experiential knowledge," i.e., through group contacts, observations, and feedback from their referrals. This, in part, was the way in which the New Jersey Self-Help Clearinghouse was initially developed—through an on-going learning experience, as staff incrementally discovered the varied benefits and growing potential of self-help. Self-help clearinghouses now offer professionals a variety of training opportunities and materials to learn more about local groups.

DEVELOPMENT OF SELF-HELP CLEARINGHOUSES

Development of the very first self-help clearinghouse in the United States was "sparked at a little committee meeting of the Lincoln Mental Health Association in the late '50s" (B. Fox, personal communication, March 8,1988). Members of the committee were involved in starting and working with programs that supported specific self-help groups. One member, who volunteered to install a telephone line to answer phone inquiries for the local Recovery self-help group, was subsequently asked to provide similar phone services for a variety of other self-help groups. This centralization led to a natural support group for self-help group leaders that, in turn, supported new initiatives and groups. In 1964, the resulting organization, that came to be known as the Self-Help Information Service of Nebraska, printed and distributed to professionals their first self-help group directory.

As more professionals have sought to tap the potential of self-help groups for prevention, as supplements to treatment, and for aftercare support, broader program initiatives have emerged. Borck and Aronowitz (1982) provide examples of the work of several early self-help centers and specify six clearinghouse responsibilities: compilation of information, provision of information and referral, technical assistance to groups and individuals, skills development training, community education, and research.

Another way of examining clearinghouse operations would be to view their goals or functions. The ten functions listed below are characteristic of most self-help clearinghouses. In reviewing these functions, it is important to understand that many agencies are already performing some of them or have existing programs that could readily address these goals to varying degrees. The functions are:

1. Increasing the identification of self-help groups through the development, distribution, and updating of listings and directories of local groups.
2. Increasing utilization of self-help groups by referring clients and clients' families to self-help groups.
3. Increasing the awareness of self-help groups on the part of the public and professional communities through publication of local listings, directories and newsletter articles; conference presentations with group representatives; and joint work with the media that educates people to the problems addressed by groups as well as the availability of groups.
4. Increasing the understanding of groups through workshops, conferences, and even staff meetings at which professionals and self-help group representatives may be provided with opportunities to "learn from one another" (President's Commission on Mental Health, 1978, p. 178). Increased understanding might also be achieved through research projects, especially joint projects that explore issues of importance and priority to groups.

5. Increasing the development of self-help groups by identifying and supporting persons who have an interest in starting new groups. By the very nature of their work, professionals are in a favorable position to identify, encourage and link current and former clients in such development efforts.
6. Increasing the networking of groups with one another and with other community resources to better meet each other's needs and to share solutions to problems. Such networking can result in needed coalitions to advocate for new services, system reform, or social change.
7. Increasing the professional interface that makes needed information, skills, and expertise more available to self-help groups that request them, while aiding professionals in understanding appropriate ways to tap self-help group resources and expertise. Examples of this interface would include professionals volunteering to serve on professional advisory committees that are maintained by some of the groups, as well as professionals inviting group representatives to participate in professional in-service training presentations or to serve on agency advisory or planning boards.
8. Helping to maintain and improve groups through direct organizational consultation to help overcome problems that may threaten group survival or to support groups in their development of special projects or service programs.
9. Providing in-kind support to self-help groups by helping to arrange for the provision of flyers, telephone services, meeting space, secretarial services, mailings, and related services.
10. Increasing advocacy for self-help groups through assistance in group coalition building, group training in self-advocacy skills, selection of group representatives for commissions and boards, and social action efforts on behalf of and with self-help groups.

Some of these functions are also performed in part by individual professionals such as clergy, physicians, or even funeral directors, but clearinghouses perform these roles in a comprehensive integrated way. The development of self-help clearinghouses has been spurred on in part by the increased recognition and growth of self-help groups in what has been described as the "self-help movement" (Gartner, & Riessman, 1977; Katz, 1981), the "prosumer" movement (Toffler, 1980), a "megatrend" (Naisbitt, 1982), or the "self-help revolution" (Gartner, & Riessman, 1984). As the number of self-help groups in the country continues to grow, it can be anticipated that mental health agencies will become increasingly involved with them. Development of self-help clearinghouse and clearinghouse-like services offers a practical program approach by which mental health agencies can create and support needed community support networks, increase understanding and collaboration between the self-help and professional communities, and address some of the mental health needs of the unserved and underserved portions of the population.

THE NEW JERSEY SELF-HELP CLEARINGHOUSE

What first began in 1978 as a small consultation and education project of a community mental health center to simply inform its own clinical staff of the availability of local community self-help groups, grew within three years into the first statewide self-help clearinghouse operation in the country. In less than seven years since its start in 1981, the New Jersey Self-Help Clearinghouse has helped to develop over five hundred new self-help groups in the state through its consultation and networking services. It currently provides self-help group referrals to over twelve thousand professional and lay callers annually over its toll-free statewide helpline. In addition to newsletters and directories, the Clearinghouse has printed a variety of how-to materials that address general issues pertaining to the development of a group as well as guidelines for starting specific types of groups such as those for manic depression, AIDS, or youth.

The center's initial contact with self-help groups began as an effort to simply identify their number and availability for referral purposes. Clinical staff had noted how helpful some groups were as supplements to treatment, citing how in some cases treatment time was reduced through their use. Groups were also meeting many emotional and practical needs that the professional staff could not address. The Consultation and Education (C&E) Department composed and distributed a one page listing of these local groups. As it was circulated both inside and outside the center, it grew to include a broad range of over seventy self-help groups for various addictions, disabilities, illnesses, parenting concerns, and other stressful life problems.

As the C&E department became known regionally for maintaining such a resource listing, staff began to receive numerous inquiries from professionals and lay persons alike who were seeking a specific support group. But in many cases no group was available. It was then that staff discovered that some "help seekers" could actually be turned into "community resource developers." This was done simply by asking callers, "Would you be interested in joining with others to develop a group?" For those who said "yes," their names were recorded so future callers, who might be interested in the same type of group, could be referred to them. Like rubbing two sticks of wood together to start a fire, those linkages with subsequent callers often resulted in the establishment of new groups.

Consultation regarding group development issues and strategies was provided to individuals who requested it, in line with the center's goals for improving the development of the community's natural support systems. In providing consultation to persons who were interested in starting a group, staff also discovered the importance of having information on, and networking with, existing national groups or one-of-a-kind model self-help groups. They observed a "demonstrational effect," wherein laypersons were more prone to start a new self-help group in their community if they could be provided with just one example of how others with their problem had actually succeeded in starting a self-help group elsewhere. They also benefited by not having to "re-invent the wheel." This led to the inclusion of national or demonstrational groups, which had no local chapters or counterparts, to the listing of self-help groups. In 1980, the listing was published as the first such directory in the state, under a grant from Hoffmann LaRoche.

In efforts to identify local groups, various national group headquarters were contacted for information on their local chapters in the county. Since their chapters were not identified by county, they sent complete listings of groups in the state. Soon the project coordinator realized that he had serendipitously accumulated a statewide database. Recognizing how the strategies, that had been learned earlier could be applied efficiently and more productively to a statewide area, a proposal was made to the State Division of Mental Health and Hospitals to develop a statewide service. The funding provided for an 800 telephone service, one staff person, and a computer. Service accessibility from any part of the state was guaranteed through the clearinghouse's toll-free telephone line. Because self-help group contacts were subject to frequent change, the computerized database was set up to maintain and expedite updating.

Computerized operations continue to provide for instantaneous retrieval of group information for callers, as well as printouts for directories. A computer software program called MASHnet has been developed which stores and retrieves self-help group information at county, regional, statewide and national levels. MASHnet, with its database of over 500 national and model groups, is used by several self-help clearinghouses in other states. The New Jersey statewide database presently contains contacts for over 3,400 group meetings in the state.

Emergence of Group Development Strategies

In initial consultations with laypersons interested in starting groups, staff responded to their frequent request for help in planning their first group meeting. While such initial group meetings were often successful, some six months later a significant number of consultees would report feeling burned out, complaining that they were still the only ones to open the church door, make the coffee, and chair the meeting. They were quite frustrated at not being able to motivate others to share responsibility for running the group. A related occurrence was that a few groups had ceased meeting after their leader, who had been a consultee of the clearinghouse, had either moved away or left the group for other reasons.

In view of these cases, brief guidelines for laypersons were drawn up which placed special emphasis on developing a core group of individuals who would agree among themselves that they would share the responsibility for developing and running the group before holding the first meeting. To establish this foundation of shared leadership, consultees were advised to first locate other persons similarly interested in starting as opposed to simply joining the group (and to phrase their publicity accordingly). In subsequent consultations, emphasis was placed on the development of this core group rather than on the first public meeting.

Results with the revised approach were excellent for those consultees who accepted the suggestion. While it took a few months longer for groups to start, fewer lay consultees reported being burned out later. An added benefit was that the more timid consultees could more easily be encouraged to take the first step in developing a group if they understood how this approach would ensure that the responsibility for group development would not be on their shoulders alone, but would be shared with others joining them in the effort. Consultees also understood how this approach of practicing mutual help from the very start would promote more active involvement on the part of all members who, from the day of the first public meeting, would see mutual help modeled for them.

In some of the first consultations with professionals, several of them indicated that they would prefer to initially lead self-help groups themselves. They planned to withdraw from the group in time, turning it over to the members. But these initial efforts rarely succeeded. In some groups, members became dependent upon the professional in a short amount of time. Some members resented the professional's leaving them. Professionals complained of members' resistance to assuming responsibilities and found themselves continuing to carry leadership tasks. One self-help group leader, who was familiar with this phenomenon, articulated the problem by noting that "serving people breakfast in bed simply doesn't give them the incentive to go to the kitchen and learn to cook breakfast for themselves." Human service professionals are by their vocation, and usually their personal inclination, very helping people. But professionals need to be aware of the unintentioned deleterious impact that they can have on a self-help group by being too helpful, e.g., doing too much for a group or providing help too soon.

Borman (1980) described the ideal professional role as an ancillary one, being "on tap but not on top." This type of approach is to serve as a consultant, wherein the professional provides advice and ideas, but does not assume responsibility for actual leadership or decision-making. As a consultant, the professional is mindful and respectful of the fact that the consultee can reject the advice that is provided. Assuming a consultant's role, and making this role clear to the consultees, can avoid many dependency and related problems. In initiating all its consultations, the Clearinghouse advises each consultee in writing as to what consultation is and how they are under no obligation to follow the suggestions provided.

For most professionals who decide to assist individuals in starting a group, the role of a group development consultant is a new one quite different from that of a clinical or case consultant. Given the skills and knowledge learned over the years, it is not easy for a professional to put them aside when attending a self-help group. While the professional often has clinical expertise related to handling the issue that the self-help group will address, this could be more of a hindrance than a help if one begins practicing within the group. Wollert, Knight and Levy (1980) note from their two-year observations of one group that many professionals tended in their first contacts to act as counselors or leaders, alienating members and undercutting the group process. Treatment professionals have a natural tendency to diagnose or psychopathologize, whereas self-help groups usually are aiming to help normalize their members, i.e., help them recognize that they are not alone, reduce their unhealthy sense of stigma, and give them a sense of how others are coping.

While professionals have to recognize how their actions might weaken self-help, they also have to begin to understand what factors might strengthen groups. Following publication of her study (1981) of both member-run self-help groups and professionally-run support groups for families of the mentally ill, Clearinghouse staff inquired of Agnes Hatfield what one characteristic she considered to be more important to the vitality of a self-help group. She responded that through her study and observations she thought it was "a sense of ownership" on the part of the members, i.e., the more the members feel it to be "their group," the more time and effort they will invest, and the more responsibility they will assume, to see that the group succeeds in its work. But when the group is perceived by members as being someone else's group, e.g., that of a professional or an agency, members will tend to be more passive and let the professional do the work. This same problem of passivity can arise when a group is perceived by its members as being run, dominated, or owned by one lay leader. The importance of member ownership, this respect and need for group autonomy, is not a new concept. Alcoholics Anonymous, which is over fifty years old, saw fit to incorporate into one of its Twelve Traditions the requirement that AA forever remain non-professional, i.e., that it be run by and for its members. The success of AA would appear to confirm the value of ownership to group vitality.

There are many other important factors that contribute to the strength of a self-help group such as ideology (Antze, 1979), or any one or combination of various outside systemic organizational supports (Leventhal, Maton & Madara, 1988) such as national affiliation, coalition membership, or agency support and endorsement. A former Clearinghouse consultant, Mariesa Julien (1988), in a survey asking 140 groups what outside support proved most helpful to them, found that the most successful of groups gained tremendous advantage by sharing with other similar groups and group leaders on a regular basis. Groups that were nationally affiliated often were already provided with such a self-help group for self-help group leaders. Based in large part on this research, the Clearinghouse increased its efforts to help self-help groups to organize both general and like-kind coalitions throughout the state. The Clearinghouse helped to form several coalitions, e.g., families of head-injured, which in time developed its own foundation and service agency. In areas where there is no self-help clearinghouse, the development of a general self-help group coalition could, as was the case in Nebraska, be a precursor to clearinghouse development.

Overview of Clearinghouse Operations and Rationale

The Clearinghouse program is divided into three primary but interdependent areas of operation: information and referral services, consultation and training services, and outreach and education services. The major goal of the Clearinghouse, and the intent of all three services, is the development of new self-help groups to meet unmet community needs for mutual aid and support. It is believed that this function, as evidenced by the large number of groups that have been started by the Clearinghouse for a wide variety of human needs, helps most to tap that potential which self-help has to offer. Also, often the development of just one new model group will subsequently result in multiple replication. One example might best illustrate this potential, a case that began when one woman called the Clearinghouse to ask if there was a group available for her post-partum depression. As there was no group to be found, she was asked by staff if she would be interested in joining with others to form such a group. She was hesitant, but later indicated she was interested after she attended a Clearinghouse conference and met representatives from several other types of groups. After her group, Depression After Delivery, was started and she appeared on one television talk show arranged through the Clearinghouse, she received a large number of requests from women and professionals in other states asking for her help in starting similar groups. She has helped to develop numerous groups and has founded an international network of post-partum depression groups, which has had several conferences and is working closely with medical professionals in reaching a better understanding of the disorder and ways in which to meet the needs of women who suffer with it.

As new problems and challenges arise in the areas of mental health, physical health, and social change, it is often self-help groups that are the first to alert the public and professional communities to the issue and the needs. As an example, the Clearinghouse in its first year of official operation, 1981, began to receive calls from persons with AIDS and a few self-help groups were subsequently started. These groups were among the first to educate the professional and lay communities—years before most professionals knew about AIDS. Similar trends took place with early calls to the Clearinghouse for other problems such as Alzheimer's Disease, caring for an elderly parent, incest, parents of troubled adolescents, and manic-depression. Early support of these groups can hasten the ongoing cycle of social change and responsive resource development in the self-help, professional, and public sectors. Because new self-help groups sometimes emerge at the cutting edge of social change, their identification and development might best be supported and accelerated by professionals, agencies, and self-help clearinghouses. For even on the local community level, groups can serve as a helpful "barometer of community stressors" (Borck & Aronowitz, 1982), shedding light on new areas of need.

A self-help clearinghouse's ability to identify and help mobilize groups dealing with new issues is important, but the majority of issues that callers present to a clearinghouse are more prevalent and common. The Clearinghouse can serve a critical resource building function by helping to develop groups for these concerns and possibly developing new model approaches in response to the felt needs of consultees. As Riessman (1984) points out, the demand for human services today far outstrips what the nation is willing to or can supply, and what is needed is a "resource building strategy that geometrically expands the help-giving potential of the society and also changes it qualitatively." A self-help clearinghouse, with development as its primary goal, can be the foundation of such a strategy.

In the first few years of the Clearinghouse, state mental health funding was increased as the demand for Clearinghouse development and information services grew. In 1985, with the help and support of self-help group representatives, state legislation was passed providing the Clearinghouse with additional general state funding that continues today. Similar state funding has enabled clearinghouse development in four other states.

This funding has allowed the Clearinghouse to grow to eight staff members. Four of these staff work in consultation, two specialize in information and referral services aided by volunteers, one coordinates outreach and education services, and a secretary assists with the development of all resource and outreach materials. With an understanding of how they can foster group development, information and referral staff help callers consider the possibility of starting a group while also linking other callers with those interested in starting groups. The outreach and education coordinator fosters group development through numerous means such as promoting newspaper media coverage of persons who are in the process of starting groups or by describing the interests of many of these same people in the Clearinghouse newsletter.

Information and Referral Service

The information and referral service helps to increase the identification and utilization of self-help groups and is usually the first contact that the public and professionals have with the Clearinghouse. Over a third of the over 12,000 annual callers are professionals. Some may call only once to learn about a particular group and subsequently use that information to make multiple patient referrals over a long period of time.

All calls are documented on the computer, which can then provide a variety of reports such as the most frequent caller requests broken down by a taxonomy of 85 major categories, the most productive sources of referrals, or the proportion of calls from each of New Jersey's twenty-one counties. Such reports can alert staff to increasing demand for groups in specific problem areas or locations, information which can help indicate future conference issues that need to be addressed or resource materials that need to be developed. Comparing call rates from different counties with their proportionate populations, staff can identify which counties have low call rates and should be targets for outreach efforts.

The Clearinghouse's database is regularly updated. Local groups are contacted at least annually for verification and updating. The questionnaire used to gather data on local groups also inquires as to how the Clearinghouse may be of further assistance to that group. In the past, returns have reflected such group needs as help with member recruitment, publicity, agency support, and fundraising. National groups are also contacted annually for updating of information on their office and local affiliates. Information on new groups is obtained through reviews of newsletters and magazines, as well as from helplines, self-help groups, an informal network of volunteers who scout prospects, and the sharing of directories and computer databases with other self-help clearinghouses.

The two information and referral staff also edit and compile an annual state directory which contains contacts for nearly four thousand local, state, national and model groups. The directory is distributed free to mental health agencies, hospitals, state agencies, and to all four hundred public libraries in the state. Under a corporate grant, a national directory (Madara & Meese, 1988) is printed every two years.

Outreach and Education Service

The outreach and education service helps to increase the awareness and understanding of self-help groups and Clearinghouse services. To educate the professional and public community to the number, diversity, and benefits of self-help groups, the Clearinghouse has used a variety of approaches, such as press releases, specialized mailings, billboards, radio and television public service announcements and programs, speaking engagements, conference displays and presentations, and a newsletter. Specialized mailings are regularly made to different professional groups, e.g., family court judges or employee health nurses, with each letter providing descriptions of relevant groups. Different outreach efforts are evaluated for effectiveness.

In response to requests for speakers, the Clearinghouse works with groups in supplying speakers for workshops, conferences, and other speaking engagements. When several speakers are requested for a particular issue, this can often provide a welcome opportunity for group representatives to explore possible coalition building or new resource development. In terms of speaking engagements of group representatives before professionals, one noteworthy observation is that five minutes of personal testimony on the part of one representative may be more effective in understanding the value and potential of self-help groups than a number of textbook readings on the subject.

Work with the media has been the primary way that the Clearinghouse has sought to bring self-help groups to public and professional attention. Staff work closely with local media in providing responses and suggestions regarding appropriate groups for particular or general articles, and in the development of regular columns or section listings of self-help groups. To maximize the impact of the increasing number of television programs and dramas depicting self-help groups, staff will often contact the media in advance of the program airing to advise them of appropriate local group contacts that could be interviewed for a timely article. While the focus for these articles has been primarily on these groups, the Clearinghouse services or telephone number are often automatically included by the media, usually at the suggestion of the self-help group representative.

In addition to the development of a weekly television call-in interview program on self-help groups which appeared on public television stations in the state, the Clearinghouse has sought to expand the impact of its work through the development of public service announcements for use by other self-help clearinghouses. Under a grant from the Prudential Foundation, television spots were developed for seven clearinghouses serving a total population of fifty million, educating viewers to the availability of groups and clearinghouses.

Consultation and Training Service

The consultation service is the main thrust of the Clearinghouse program. There are a number of resources that the Clearinghouse draws upon to accomplish this work. Using the same taxonomy as the information service, hundreds of how-to materials are gleaned, obtained, and compiled as a result of contacts with groups and regular review of their newsletters and publications. Newspaper articles that exemplify personal successes in group development are similarly filed and subsequently distributed to encourage those who may be considering group development. Handouts on general steps and strategies for both laypersons and those professionals interested in group development (Madara & Meese, 1986, pp. 101-108) are provided to new consultees, along with information on specific national and model groups and their group development guidelines. A range of other how-to materials have been developed to provide consultees with general suggestions on such topics as member recruitment, group discussion, meeting formats, and finding a meeting place.

A key resource in the development of both general and specific guidelines has been interviews with self-help group representatives and materials obtained from their groups. Staff also visit groups that are open to visitors in order to observe the diversity and dynamics of different group approaches. As Silverman (1980) points out, of the many ways that a professional can learn about self-help groups, "the most effective is to learn from existing mutual help groups." All Clearinghouse staff have an ongoing responsibility for such learning and are required to make regular visits to open groups in line with guidelines that respect group autonomy and dynamics (Wollert, Knight, & Levy, 1980).

The Clearinghouse augments its staff through the use of self-help group representatives as paid consultants. While the growth of self-help is based in good part on the volunteer efforts of veterans of established groups who contribute their time and energy to help potential leaders develop new groups in other geographic areas, there are situations where financial, distance, group focus differences, or other constraints make it difficult or impossible for this help to be provided naturally. In such situations where support would not otherwise be provided, the Clearinghouse provides travel and conference reimbursement to consultees and payment to group consultants in order to enable individuals who are starting groups to receive advice, suggestions, training, and related consultation from veterans who are familar with the problems, pitfalls and successful strategies involved. Consultation is provided primarily over the phone, an ideal medium that allows support to be provided while lessening the risk of consultee over-dependence on the consultant that is sometimes possible with face-to-face consults. Conferences and workshops are held throughout the state to provide training in the development of new groups, help on issues of current concern to existing groups, and to highlight new types of groups and group approaches. The Clearinghouse seeks out opportunities to present at other state conferences, from those for school psychologists to those for home economists. The spectrum of potential community helpers who can assist and encourage people to develop groups is extremely broad and multidisciplinary, from clergy to community service organizations like Junior League. Conferences are taped for later use by consultees or for general public or professional education.

The Clearinghouse has sought to maintain a proactive approach to group development that goes beyond simply being responsive to requests for consultation. Examples of proactive efforts are outreach to agencies and communities to demonstrate new out-of-state group models to serve a particular population in need, development of new how-to materials dealing with issues for which there are few self-help group models or materials, outreach to and coordination with national self-help groups dealing with prevalent issues for which there are few or no groups in the state, and the development and funding of specialty programs for populations that are unserved or underserved by self-help. Eleven criteria used by the Clearinghouse to determine target populations or groups are the number of unmet requests by callers for these groups, the number of current consultees seeking assistance in developing this type of group, the prevalence of problem or concern, the incidence or growth rate of the problem, a lack of professional resources directed to the issue, a lack of a national self-help group dealing with issue, a lack of group models for the issue, a lack of existing how-to resource materials for group development, the severity of the problem, the degree to which the problem isolates or alienates persons with it, and the appropriateness of the self-help modality for ameliorating the problem through support, education, and advocacy efforts. These criteria were helpful in planning the first how-to guides in the country focused upon starting self-help groups for persons with AIDS, manic depression, and rare illness. Examples of other proactive efforts vary from approaching a university's osteoporosis treatment center with information on successful groups started in Canada, resulting in the first self-help group in the United States for the condition being started, to contacting community activists in Lyme, Connecticut, to advise them of the Clearinghouse's availability to help persons in New Jersey organize Lyme disease support groups, resulting in the development of the first group. The Clearinghouse has also sponsored several initiatives to examine and promote minority self-help groups and needs. In these and similar ways, clearinghouses can begin to realize their full potential for proactively addressing human needs in their communities.

Clearinghouse efforts have resulted in the development of separately funded programs to develop groups for specific populations. In 1982, with funding from the State Division of Mental Health and Hospitals, the Clearinghouse started a three year program focused on the development of groups for mental health consumers and for families of mental patients. A unique component of the program that took into account the general low income level of the population, was the provision of technical assistance mini-grants to newly started groups that planned, proposed, and used their members to carry out special service projects. Modeled upon a Self-Help Neighborhood Awards Program (SNAP) that the author had worked with in New York City neighborhoods, the program enabled unincorporated groups to develop projects such as member-run helplines, newsletters, and, in one case, the repair of a donated van to meet the travel needs of members. After the development of the groups, both consumer and family groups formed their own respective coalitions and received state funding.

A similar program was started in 1984, with funding from the State Commission for the Blind, to develop self-help groups for persons who were losing their sight or were blind. The program originated when one caller to the Clearinghouse, who was blind himself, pointed out the need for such a project. Subsequently, he became the program coordinator and, with the aid of another consultant who is also blind, has helped to develop over thirty new self-help groups throughout the state. Their work has revealed the special mental health needs of persons experiencing this disability.

Other specialty programs have included a Federal VISTA volunteer project that worked in the development of self-help groups for youth and produced a how-to development manual on the subject. Other how-to manuals have focused on starting groups for families of the mentally ill, for those who are unemployed seeking jobs, and for smoking cessation.

EMPOWERMENT VERSUS ENFEEBLEMENT

A few examples of how professionals can strengthen or weaken groups, the latter often done inadvertently, have been presented. Borman (1979) described how in the past it has been maverick professionals, i.e., those working outside the mainstream of their discipline, who played key roles in developing, supporting, and empowering self-help groups. But over the past few years, the interest in and interface with self-help has expanded from individual professionals to the level of agencies, institutions, and government. With the involvement of more agencies and institutions, the interface between self-help groups and professionals has become more formal and bureaucratic. Some see this as the threat of professionalization or colonization (Wilson, 1986). Such a threat remains real if professionals fail to learn and understand the values, principles, and dynamics of self-help groups. In very positive ways, self-help groups empower people and help them to regain control of their lives, rather than having their lives controlled by an addiction, disability, loss, or stressful life event. Individuals realize what they can do for themselves, for others in the group and, in some cases, what their groups can achieve through joint advocacy. Professionals have a real role in respecting and supporting those empowerment efforts for the ultimate benefit of their patients and communities. The future of the interface between self-help groups and professionals will largely be determined by the degree to which professionals become better educated to the distinctive benefits that member-run self-help groups provide and understand the most appropriate professional and agency roles to develop, promote, and support these groups. Self-help clearinghouses and similar projects can serve as models to help maximize the potential that exists for synergistic relationships that improve community mental health.

PERSPECTIVES ON ADDITIONAL SELF-HELP TRENDS

As self-help groups continue to grow, there are some trends that may be noted within the larger self-help megatrend (Naisbitt, 1982). The first perspective may be gained by examining the past to anticipate the future. Historically the seeds for the development of many long-standing health foundations, societies, and agencies dealing with various individual illnesses or social concerns have first taken the form of self-help groups or networks. These community support services were created by persons with the disorder and/or their families as they networked with one another and became aware of their common needs and their abilities to help one another through group support and action. Some examples include parents of the mentally retarded organizing in the 1950s to eventually form the Association for Retarded Children, Marjorie Guthrie pulling together other families to form what today is the Huntington's Disease Society of America, and Sylvia Lawry, whose brother had multiple sclerosis, eventually founding the Multiple Sclerosis Society from initial patient and family meetings she arranged through an ad she placed in a local newspaper.

This cycle continues today. As relatively new health problems, syndromes, addictions, and chronic disorders arise or increase in prevalence, e.g., Alzheimer's or AIDS, it is often the self-help networks that are the first to provide support, information, skills sharing, education of professionals, and needed advocacy. This is especially true when existing institutions are not aware of or sensitive to these needs, in which case groups may advocate and work towards development of a new service organization of their own.

A factor contributing to this current trend in the health field is improved medical technology and research, which continues to increase the survival and prevalence rates for previously life-threatening injuries and disorders while continuing to identify new specialty disorders and syndromes. The result is that more children are now born with disabilities than in prior times. Also, the increase in longevity and the greying of the population is causing a proportionate increase in the prevalence of chronic and disabling conditions.

The health care system has succeeded in saving and prolonging life with serious chronic illness or disability but has failed to provide the needed psychosocial support to help the increasing number of survivors and their families who must cope with the demands and stress. Mental health agencies can be expected to see more individuals and families that are facing these stresses. In addition, another cluster of self-help groups has arisen simply to deal with the iatrogenic or ill effects of medicine, e.g., DES Mothers and Daughters, the Dalkon Shield Network, and DPT—Dissatisfied Parents Together (parents of children with adverse reactions to DPT shots). A number of other self-help groups have been developed just to deal with environmental illnesses, such as the Association of Birth Defect Children (due to environmental agents), the White Lung Association (asbestos victims), the Brown Lung Association (cotton textile workers), and the Human Ecology Action League. To meet the needs of an increasing portion of the population suffering from a chronic, genetic, rare, environmental, or iatrogenic illness, new self-help organizations will continue to be needed to provide initial and ongoing support, education, and advocacy. In the area of rare disorders alone, the Clearinghouse has helped a large number of individuals in the development of new self-help organizations. Many more groups and new support networks could be developed in other states and on a national basis if encouragement and support were available.

In the immediate future, more national attention can be expected to be drawn to self-help groups through the efforts of U.S. Surgeon General Koop who, in 1987, sponsored a national Surgeon General's Workshop on Self-Help and Public Health to explore how self-help groups and health care professionals could work together for the benefit of public health. Among the Workshop recommendations that Dr. Koop has already enacted has been the development of a National Council on Self-Help and Public Health which will work to increase the awareness, utilization, and understanding of self-help groups on a national level. Also, as a result of initial meetings at the Workshop, a number of self-help groups subsequently met in New Jersey and formed the first national alliance of self-help groups, SHALL. The Self-Help Alliance will serve as a support organization for national self-help groups and intends to plan programs that promote the principles, practices, and philosophies of self-help as a means of empowerment.

In a 1984 national Louis Harris poll (Macro Systems, 1985) of 2,387 adults, 3% of the sample said they were currently participating in a self-help group, an additional 5% said they had participated in the past year, and 91% indicated they had never been involved. Given the wide variety of stressful life transitions that each and every person experiences in life, plus the prevalence of addictions, abuse, illness, divorce, parenting problems, and many other stressful life events, self-help groups offer outstanding potential for helping a much greater percentage of the population to better cope with stress, pain, and adversity—if there are the local resources and strategies to develop and maximize that potential.

A final trend is in its infancy but shows considerable potential for the future of self-help. It is the use of high-tech resources to create new self-help networks. In recent years some groups, such as those for mental health consumers, have been exploring the use of telephone conference calls as an effective means of networking over great distances. A few self-help groups that have difficulty in meeting in traditional face-to-face communities are now meeting via home computer teleconferences. Through national computer information systems, whereby persons using their home computer can access a national system by dialing a local telephone number, discussion forums are accessible at all hours of the day and night via computer-phone linkages. Questions, information, and messages can be left on a bulletin board for others to respond to. Actual conference meetings take place on-line. Regularly scheduled Alcoholics Anonymous meetings are attended by members from their homes. Members type their remarks as the comments of all other members scroll up from the bottom of the computer screen. Persons who are both deaf and blind facilitate weekly self-help group meetings for persons with disabilities. Persons who have a rare illness, but are separated by thousands of miles, are provided with their first opportunity to share with others who have their disorder and to compare experiences. Terminally ill cancer patients from their hospice beds can share their fears and insights using portable computers. These are just a few examples of ways in which technology is providing a new dimension to self-help communities.

On one national system called CompuServe, the Clearinghouse has assisted the development of several self-help group meetings, e.g., one for persons with multiple sclerosis and another for persons with Ehlers Danlos Syndrome. Since their first meeting, several of the persons with Ehlers Danlos Syndrome formed their own national foundation, the first of its type in the country. The Clearinghouse has also hosted a national meeting for agoraphobics with the founder of Agoraphobics Anonymous as the guest speaker. As computer equipment becomes both more affordable and better integrated into routine phone communications, more individuals, families and groups may take advantage of this medium for mutual support, information sharing, and conferencing.

CONCLUSION

Self-help groups continue to increase in number and diversity in response to felt needs for peer support, practical information, coping skills, and needed advocacy efforts on the part of individuals and families. In addition to serving as viable supports for the prevention of stress and dysfunction in the community, groups can supplement treatment services, provide long-term aftercare support, promote public relations, and serve as helpful allies in advocacy efforts for needed services, funding, and research. With the increased national attention and growth, there will be more occasions and opportunities for mental health agencies to work with, support, and develop self-help groups for the benefit of their own patients and local communities. One important way in which agencies and clearinghouses alike can tap the rich resource-building potential of self-help is to simply identify, encourage, and link persons who are potential group founders. But there are a variety of principles, such as respect for group autonomy and ownership, that should be understood and practiced in order to avoid potential pitfalls. By tapping the resources of existing self-help clearinghouses, or through the development of clearinghouse-like consultation, referral, and outreach and education services, mental health agencies can help other professionals, agencies, and the public to maximize the use and development of these community supports to promote competence, prevent dependency, ameliorate illness-producing life stress, and address social problems and system failures that contribute to human suffering.

REFERENCES

Albee, G.W. (1982). Preventing psychopathology and promoting human potential. *American Psychologist*, *37* (9), 1043-1050.

Antze, P. (1979). Role of ideologies in peer psychotherapy groups. In M. A. Lieberman & L.D. Borman (Eds.), *Self-help groups for coping with crisis* (pp. 272-304). San Francisco: Jossey-Bass.

Black, R.B. & Drachman, D. (1985). Hospital social workers and self-help groups. *Health and Social Work*, *10* (2), 95-103.

Borck, L.E. & Aronowitz, E. (1982). The role of the self-help clearinghouse. In L. D. Borman, L.E. Borck, R. Hess, & F.L. Pasquale (Eds.), *Helping people to help themselves: Self-help and prevention* (pp. 121-129). New York: Haworth.

Borman, L. D. (1979). Characteristics of development and growth. In M.A. Lieberman & L.D. Borman (Eds.). *Self-help groups for coping with crisis*. San Francisco: Jossey-Bass.

Borman, L.D. (1980). The professional as facilitator: Helping self-help groups help themselves. *D.D. Polestar*, newsletter Developmental Disabilities Training Systems and Technical Resource Center-Region II, *1* (9), 7.

Borman, L.D. & Lieberman, M.A. (1979). Conclusion: Contributions, dilemmas, and implications for mental health policy. In M.A. Lieberman & L.D. Borman (Eds.) *Self-help groups for coping with crisis*. San Francisco: Jossey-Bass.

Chamberlin, J. (1978). *On our own: Patient-controlled alternatives to the mental health system*. New York: McGraw-Hill.

Chutis, L. (1983). Special roles of mental health professionals in self-help group development. *Prevention in Human Services*, *2*, 65-73.

Gartner, A., & Riessman, F. (1977). *Self-help in the human services*. San Francisco: Jossey-Bass.

Gartner, A., & Riessman, F. (Eds.). (1984). *The self-help revolution*. New York: Human Sciences.

Giloth, B. (1981, November). *Hospital involvement with self help/support groups*. Paper presented at the annual meeting of the American Public Health Association.

Hatfield, A.B. (1981). Self-help groups for the families of the mentally ill. *Social Work*, *26* (5), 408-413.

Hess, R. (1980). Helping thyself to mental health: An interview. *Innovation*, 7, 18-21.

Jeger, A.M., Slotnick, R.S., & Schure, M. (1982). Towards a "self-help/professional collaborative model" of mental health service delivery. In D.E. Biegel, & A. J. Naperstek (Eds.), *Community support systems and mental health: Practice, policy and research* (pp. 205-223). New York: Springer.

Julien, T. M. (1988) *The relationship between self-help groups and the community organizations that provide their resources*. Doctoral dissertation, Teachers College, Columbia University.

Katz, A.H. (1981). Self-help and mutual aid: An emerging social movement? *Annual Review of Sociology*, 7, 129-155.

Katz, A. H., & Hermalin, J. (1987). Self-help and prevention. In J. Hermalin & J. A. Morell (Eds.), *Prevention planning in mental health* (pp. 151-190). Beverly Hills: Sage Publications.

Leventhal, G.S., Maton, M.I., & Madara, E.J. (1988). Systemic organizational support for self-help groups. *American Journal of Orthopsychiatry 58* (4), 592-603.

Macro Systems, Inc. (1985). *A study of the sources, correlates, and manifestations of perceived and experienced stress in the United States*. Springfield, Virginia: National Technical Information Center. (NTIS No. PB 86-178878)

Madara, E. J. (1985). The self-help clearinghouse operation: Tapping the resource development potential of I & R Services. *Information and Referral*, *8* (1), 42-58.

Madara, E. J. (1986). A comprehensive systems approach to promoting mutual aid self-help groups. *Journal of Voluntary Action Research*, *15* (2), 57-63.

Madara, E. J. (1987). Supporting self-help: A clearinghouse perspective. *Social Policy*, *18* (2), 28-29.

Madara, E.J. & Meese, A. (1986). *The self-help sourcebook: Finding and forming mutual aid self-help groups*. Denville, New Jersey: St. Clares-Riverside Medical Center.

Naisbitt, J. (1982). *Megatrends*: New York: Warner Books.
Parents Anonymous. (1976, Winter). *Parents Anonymous Frontiers Newsletter*. (Available from Parents Anonymous, 6733 South Sepulaveda, Los Angeles, CA 90045).
President's Commission on Mental Health. (1978). *Report to the president from the President's Commission on Mental Health*. Task panel reports, (Vol. 2). Washington, DC: U.S. Government Printing Office.
Riessman, F. (1965). The helper therapy principle. *Social Work, 10*, 26-32.
Riessman, F. (1984, June). *Support groups as preventive intervention*. Paper presented at Vermont Conference on Primary Prevention of Psychopathology, Burlington.
Silverman, P.R. (1978). *Mutual help groups: A guide for mental health workers*. (DHHS Publication No. ADM 80-646) Rockville, Maryland: National Institute of Mental Health.
Silverman, P.R. (1980). *Mutual help groups: Organization and development*, Beverly Hills: Sage.
Silverman, P.R. (1985). Tertiary/secondary prevention—preventive intervention: the case for mutual help groups. In R.K. Conyne (Ed.), *The group workers' handbook* (pp237-258). Springfield, Illinois: Charles C. Thomas.
Swift, C. (1979). Report of the council on prevention. *National Council of Community Mental Health Centers annual report*. Washington, DC: NCCMHC.
Toffler, A. (1980). *The third wave*. New York: William Morrow & Co.
U.S. Department of Health & Human Services. (1980). *Promoting health/prevention disease: Objectives for the nation*. Washington, DC: U.S. Government Printing Office.
U.S. Department of Health & Human Services. (1986). *The 1990 health objectives for the nation: A midcourse review*. Washington, DC: U.S. Government Printing Office.
Wilson, J. (1986, March). *The self-help parade*. Paper presented at Association of Researchers in Voluntary Action and Community Involvement Conference, London.
Wollert, R. (1985). An information and referral model for improving community utilization of self-help groups. *Information and Referral*, 7 (2), 1-16.
Wollert, R.W., & Barron, N. (1983). Avenues of collaboration. In D.L. Pancoast, P. Parker, & C. Froland (Eds.), *Rediscovering self-help: Its role in social care* (pp. 105-123). Beverly Hills: Sage.
Wollert, R.W., Knight, B. & Levy, L.H. (1980). Make today count: a collaborative model for professionals and self-help groups. *Professional Psychology, 11* (1), 130-138.
Wollert, R. & Self-Help Research Team. (1987). The self-help clearinghouse concept: An evaluation of one program and its implications for policy and practice. *American Journal of Community Psychology, 14* (4), 491-508.